Hitting the Road

A GUIDE TO TRAVEL NURSING

HITTING THE ROAD

A Guide to Travel Nursing

Shalon Kearney, RN, MSN, CNOR
Santa Rosa, California

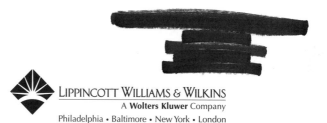

LIPPINCOTT WILLIAMS & WILKINS
A **Wolters Kluwer** Company
Philadelphia • Baltimore • New York • London
Buenos Aires • Hong Kong • Sydney • Tokyo

Acquisitions Editor: Alan Sorkowitz
Editorial Assistant: Daniel Pepper
Senior Project Editor: Rosanne Hallowell
Senior Production Manager: Helen Ewan
Managing Editor / Production: Erika Kors

Art Director: Carolyn O'Brien
Manufacturing Manager: William Alberti
Indexer: Vicki Boyle
Printer: Data Reproductions Corporation

9 8 7 6 5 4 3 2 1

Library of Congress Cataloging-in-Publication Data

Kearney, Shalon
   Hitting the road: a guide to travel nursing/Shalon Kearney.
      p. cm.
   Includes bibliographical references and index.
   ISBN 0-7817-3941-1
      1. Nursing. 2. Nursing—Miscellanea. 3. Travel—Health aspects. I. Title.

RT50.5 .K43 2003
610.73—dc21

2002022733

Care has been taken to confirm the accuracy of the information presented and to describe generally accepted practices. However, the author and publisher are not responsible for errors or omissions or for any consequences from application of the information in this book and make no warranty, express or implied, with respect to the content of the publication.

The author and publisher have exerted every effort to ensure that drug selection and dosage set forth in this text are in accordance with the current recommendations and practice at the time of publication. However, in view of ongoing research, changes in government regulations, and the constant flow of information relating to drug therapy and drug reactions, the reader is urged to check the package insert for each drug for any change in indications and dosage and for added warnings and precautions This is particularly important when the recommended agent is a new or infrequently employed drug.

Some drugs and medical devices presented in this publication have Food and Drug Administration (FDA) clearance for limited use in restricted research settings. It is the responsibility of the health care provider to ascertain the FDA status of each drug or device planned for use in his or her clinical practice.

LWW.com

This book is dedicated to
all my fellow travelers.

Preface

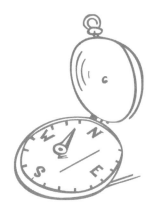

For years I toured the countryside as a "traveling nurse." I stumbled along figuring things out as I went. It wasn't until my second year of traveling that I realized how much I had learned about traveling and how much there was to know. After this realization, I felt a little frustrated that my learning had been so inefficient. If only someone could have told me these things in the beginning...I would have planned differently and thus benefited even more from my travel experiences. For example, it wasn't until the end of my sixth assignment that I discovered the benefit of collecting receipts for food expenses and deducting them from my taxes at the end of the year. Often, I thought someone should write a book for health care travelers. It would have been so helpful to have known the ins and outs from the beginning.

Later I stopped traveling and went back to school for my graduate degree in nursing. Soon after graduating, I was back on the road again. I took an assignment in Alaska for the summer along with several other travelers. Surprisingly, I found that nothing had changed: travelers were still grasping for information and resources. This time, however, I had some of the answers.

That is when I decided to write *Hitting the Road: A Guide to Travel Nursing*. At first, I wasn't sure there would be enough to write about, so I started writing about anything that came to mind regarding traveling. Soon the subject matter took on a life of its own and grew into a book for travelers. The subject, the energy, and the need were already there. I simply helped shape it and put it in legible form to benefit all travelers.

Much of the information in this book is based on 9 years of personal experience with agency nursing, and contributions from other experienced health care travelers who were excited about sharing their knowledge with you. Although much of the content is addressed to the nursing profession, any health care professional can benefit from the information and resources provided here.

Hitting the Road discusses topics ranging from how to enter the travel profession to traveling abroad. Chapters 1 through 4 discuss the concept of travel nursing, and include exercises to help you assess your travel goals and explore ways to overcome perceived obstacles. A realistic perspective regarding the advantages and disadvantages of travel nursing is presented, along with accounts of some real-life travel experiences. (*Note:* Except where identified otherwise, the names of the travelers cited through the book have been changed to protect their privacy.) Chapters 5 through 9 discuss the more practical aspects of travel nursing, such as how to prepare for the application process, get the assignment you desire, negotiate a travel contract, and organize your travel. You learn the important questions to ask while talking with staffing companies, which documents to have in place, which benefits are negotiable and which ones are not, what to ask during a hospital interview, what is tax deductible and what is not, and much more. Chapter 10 briefly discusses international travel nursing. Finally, the Appendices offer resources on travel nursing; state licensure information; a list of volunteer organizations; and information on 70 health care staffing agencies in the United States to use as a guide in finding your perfect assignment.

Now, health care professionals have the opportunity to benefit from the experiences of other professional travelers everywhere. This compilation of helpful hints, agency information and anecdotal advice will help travelers to earn the most while minimizing "beginner's" mistakes. By the time you finish reading this book, you will have a good idea of what health care travel is really like and whether it would be right for you. You will be able to enter the profession with insight and clarity. If you are an experienced traveler, you will enjoy reading about other travelers' experiences, learn how to maximize your income with tax deductions, and have more resources at your fingertips for both domestic and international travel.

This book is an exciting step toward bringing travelers together as a group and acknowledging them as a professional niche requiring unique skills and knowledge. By sharing information and knowledge, we can play a part in shaping the future of the expanding health care travel industry.

Shalon Kearney, RN, MSN, CNOR

Acknowledgments

I would like to acknowledge the following people, without whose help completing this book would have been a much more difficult task:

- Jazmine Canfield—for being a wonderful mother and allowing me to stay at her place between assignments for 3 months while I began writing this book.
- Ken Williams—for editing a chapter for me in the beginning stages.
- Mark Hernandez—for spending many late nights at various Internet cafes working on projects while I wrote my book, and for reading my book and providing much valuable input throughout its creation.
- Austin Writers' League—for consistently critiquing my work and making me feel like my book was not only a good idea, but also possible.
- Anna Mari Lilja—for editing some of my work and suggesting several times that I make writing a priority if I wanted to finish the book. (Finally, I got the message and began a disciplined writing schedule.)
- Chris Ransom—for always sharing new travel information.
- Charlotte Culpepper, Patricia Tubin, Penny Nichols, Tony Trusty II, Denise Calhoun, Margaret Washburn, Paul Baker, Kim Groves, Brian Salensky, Chris Ransom, Pam Mularcik—for sharing their travel experiences and allowing me to share them with you.
- Mindy Reed—for editing my first official draft to present to the publisher.
- Gina Katigbak—for being a supportive and encouraging friend and having so much faith in me.
- Chet Kearney—for being a wonderful father. Thanks for driving me an hour to meet my publisher.
- Alan Sorkowitz—for being a patient and thorough editor.

Contents

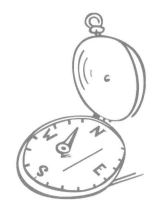

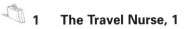

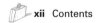

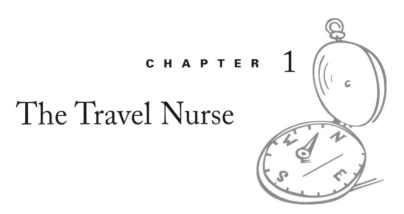

CHAPTER 1

The Travel Nurse

Before discussing the pursuits of a professional traveler, the term *traveler* must be defined in the context of the health care profession today. Travelers come in all shapes and sizes, and they travel for a variety of reasons. Much diversity exists, but travelers share similar characteristics that draw them to the traveling profession. These similarities often allow travelers to bond easily with one another.

WHO ARE TRAVELERS?

Travelers are health professionals who contract their patient care services through a professional staffing agency in hospitals nationwide and abroad. Contracts are for a designated length of time (usually 3 months) at one particular facility.

WHO ESTABLISHES THE CONTRACTS?

Professional staffing agencies (also referred to in this book as "travel agencies") negotiate contracts with hospitals in the United States and other countries. These staffing agencies are independent from any structured health facilities.

WHAT TYPE OF PEOPLE DO AGENCIES LOOK FOR?

Agencies look for experienced professionals, and the more experienced, the better. The demand is higher for specialty areas, and certifications are helpful. Generally, agencies require a minimum of 12 months' experience in the desired specialty.

Recruiters stress the importance of people skills. When a hospital terminates a contract, it is usually because the traveler did not get along well with others in the facility, not because of lack of technical skill. Therefore, recruiters feel better about sending travelers who are team players, outgoing, prompt, and professional.

While all these characteristics are important, the quality that agencies most prefer from travelers is flexibility. The fewer limits you set, the easier it is for the agency to find you work. If you are too flexible, however, you may find yourself in a less than desirable situation. Try to be flexible, but stand your ground on issues that are important to you. This book will help you clarify your goals so that you can negotiate for what you want while being flexible on the rest.

WHAT AREAS OF EXPERTISE ARE REQUIRED TO TRAVEL?

Opportunities to travel are available to several different types of health care professionals.

Nurses can travel within specialty areas:
- Operating Room (OR)
- Intensive Care Unit (ICU)
- Critical Care Unit (CCU)
- Neonatal Intensive Care Unit (NICU)
- Emergency Room (ER)
- Psychiatry
- Midwife Telemetry
- Pediatrics (PEDS) Medical/Surgical (MS)
- Labor and Delivery (L&D)
- Correctional facilities

Nurses from different degree programs can travel:
- Registered Nurse First Assistant (RNFA)
- Licensed Vocational Nurse (LVN)
- Licensed Practical Nurse (LPN)
- Certified Nurse Anesthetist (CRNA)
- Nurse Practitioner (NP)

Additional health care professionals can travel:
- Rehabilitation Therapist
- Respiratory Therapist (RT)
- Occupational Therapist (OT)
- Speech Pathologist (SLP)
- Pharmacist
- Radiology Technician
- Physical Therapist
- Surgical Technologist (ST)
- Biomedical Information Technologist
- Medical Technologist
- Doctors (MD)

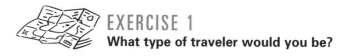

EXERCISE 1
What type of traveler would you be?

Travelers have many different reasons for traveling, but one particular reason will dominate over the others. Some professionals travel to avoid burnout. Others travel to see the world, broaden their professional experience, visit family, relocate, or simply to get away. One nurse says she travels to pay her mortgage. She has a nice house on a remote island, and traveling allows her to make more money and enjoy her house between assignments.

Look over the following types of travelers and circle the one that best describes you. Being as honest with yourself as possible will help you be clear about your goals. When you are clear about your goals, you will be clear about your choices.

The Adventurous Traveler
You love to see and do as much in life as possible. The thought of going to a new place is exciting. You adore new experiences and live in the moment.

The Financial Traveler
You focus on making things happen. Your goal is to pay off any debts and invest in a sound future. You may find yourself saying, "Show me the money."

The Empty Nest Traveler
You are looking for a way to deal with the anxiety of your children leaving home. Until now, they have taken up a considerable amount of your time. You want to make use of this extra time by doing something you want to do.

The Nonpolitical Traveler
What you dislike most about your workplace is the politics involved. You often wish you could just go to work, do your job, and not have to worry about all the bureaucracy. Being a "temporary visitor" to a workplace is appealing to you.

The Reviving Traveler
Sometimes you find yourself wondering why you got into health care in the first place. You no longer feel challenged by your work,

continued

exercise 1 continued

yet you feel more tired than ever before. The idea of adding variety to your work and learning new things sounds refreshing.

The Relocating Traveler

You are moving to a new place soon. You are not sure where you want to work when you get there, but you would like to have a job lined up already. You want to make the transition as smooth as possible.

The Independent Traveler

You want more control of your time. You are tired of dictated vacation and holiday schedules. You do not want to be on call at whim. The idea of making these decisions for yourself is empowering and desirable.

The Career-Oriented Traveler

You want to be one of the best in your profession, marketable and in demand. The idea of working in some of the best facilities in the country or the world is appealing. You often feel that working at the same place limits your professional growth.

SELF EVALUATION: SHOULD YOU BECOME A HEALTH CARE TRAVELER?

You may have more of an idea by now whether you can travel and why you want to travel. You may still wonder if traveling is for you, however. Would you be happy as a traveler? Do you have what it takes to be a traveler?

Although health professionals from all walks of life and situations travel, they do appear to have similar characteristics. Traveling, by nature, tends to attract a particular kind of person.

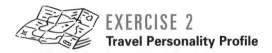

EXERCISE 2
Travel Personality Profile

This questionnaire will help you determine whether the traveling profession and your personality style are a desirable match. Choose the answer that best describes you most of the time.

1. In the face of change you:
   a. Like to roll with the punches.
   b. Like plenty of notice so you can plan ahead.

continued

exercise 2 continued

2. At this stage in your life, which do you value more?
   a. The stability of a home
   b. Experiencing new and different things
3. Do you prefer:
   a. The unknown
   b. The known
4. When faced with new situations you tend to:
   a. Need time to adjust.
   b. Adapt quickly.
5. In unknown situations, you think it is best to:
   a. Jump in and figure it out as you go.
   b. Wait for instructions.
6. Would you describe yourself as more:
   a. Disorganized
   b. Organized
7. When faced with a challenge, you first look for:
   a. A solution by yourself.
   b. Outside help.
8. How would you describe yourself?
   a. Get homesick easily.
   b. Free spirited.

Now go back over the test and count all the even-numbered questions to which you answered "A." Write down the total. Now go back and count all the odd-numbered items to which you answered "B." Add the number to your "A total" to get your overall score.

Even-numbered "A" responses _____

Odd-numbered "B" responses _____

Overall total _____

Would you be a happy health care traveler? If you overall score is above 6, it is likely that you would *not* like traveling. If your total score is between 4 and 6, you may not like traveling as much (or as often) as you think. Try working for a local agency to get an idea of the flexibility required for traveling. Then, if all goes well, try a travel assignment or two to see how and if you adjust. If your total score is between 1 and 3, then you probably will enjoy traveling from the start. In fact, you probably already know it is something you want to do.

People who enjoy travel tend to be adventurous, flexible, independent, organized, friendly, assertive, and enjoy challenge.

continued

exercise 2 continued

Now, assume you know you want to be a health care traveler, but you are still hesitant to take the first step. This reaction is normal. Taking the first step is the most difficult part.

Before you read any further, please do the following exercises to become clear on whether or not you want to travel professionally and what kind of experience you desire.

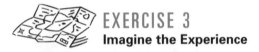

EXERCISE 3
Imagine the Experience

Set a timer, and take 5 minutes to imagine the most ideal experience of being a traveling health care traveler.

- Where do you go and why?
- Imagine you are really there.
- What kind of place are you working in?
- Are you traveling alone?
- What do you do with your time off?
- Are you working days, evenings, or nights?

Visualize as many details as possible. Write them down so you can actually see what you expect from traveling. How do you feel after imagining the travel experience?

Create whatever life you desire. You will be given choices of where to go, where to work, and what shift to work. You do not have to settle for less than what you desire.

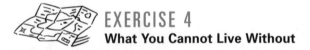

EXERCISE 4
What You Cannot Live Without

From the previous exercise, when you imagined being a health care traveler, write down all the things your imagination enjoyed. Then cross off as many as you can until you are left with only a few that you would have trouble living without. Keep these few items in mind when you are looking for an assignment and creating your future.

One of the best benefits of traveling is the variety of choices that open up to you. You can now think about your future in new and exciting ways.

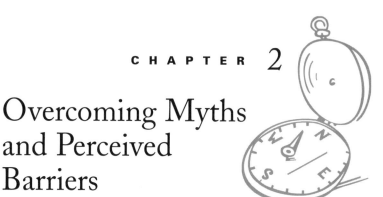

CHAPTER 2

Overcoming Myths and Perceived Barriers

One of the biggest reasons health care professionals might not pursue travel opportunities when they should is because of unspoken expectations and criteria taken for granted as truth. After all, these perceived "rules" seem logical. If you want to follow your desire, however, take a closer look at the logic. The truth is that many of the unspoken criteria for traveling are myths. Let's take a closer look.

Myth 1: Traveling Is for Young People

Absolutely not! Age is not a barrier for the traveler. Actually, agency recruiters are seeking mature and experienced nurses. Women in their sixties have been known to travel extensively. Most people who travel late in life only wish they had started sooner. Many travel when it is time to retire and the kids are grown. One major firm reports the average age of a traveling nurse to be 36.3 years (Dull, 1999).

Myth 2: Traveling Is for Single People

Another common myth about traveling is that traveling is for single people. One nurse, Rebecca, said that her husband was not interested in traveling with her. "Have you ever heard of a nurse who travels and leaves her husband at home?" she asked.

The answer is "yes." Individual situations are different, but many married people travel separately. For example, a traveler named Mary goes to Alaska every summer. She leaves her family for her own summer adventure and returns to spend the rest of the year at home.

Another traveler, Beth, travels and her husband comes to visit her. Beth says her husband loves having a place he can visit her, because "It is like we are dating all over again."

Myth 3: Traveling Is for Full-Time Nomads

Possibilities allow you to create your own options. Traveling does not have to be all or nothing. Some travelers work per diem in their hometown, and then travel in the winter. You too can balance family, friends, and adventure.

Myth 4: Traveling Is Not for Pet Owners

Many travelers bring their pets. Pets make great travel companions. It is a little more difficult for the agency to find housing for travelers with pets, but they can do it. You may be responsible for paying a pet deposit, however. If the agency is hesitant to cooperate with your request, simply switch agencies. Many agencies are "pet friendly."

Myth 5: Traveling Is Not for Mothers

Many mothers figure out ways to travel. For example, home schooling her 16-year-old son allows one 46-year-old mother to travel with him. Mary, a mother of eight children, travels to provide for her family. Sometimes the family stays at home, but sometimes they travel with her. "I took my family to Seattle one year," Mary says. "During my phone interview, I made sure it was an assignment that I could extend over the next year. We left in the summer before school started and loved it. I can't believe how many travelers there are with children. I thought I would be the minority."

Myth 6: Traveling Is for Those Excited About Their Profession

Actually, travel nursing is recommended to anyone who is feeling in a rut. Some think the answer is a career change, but most do not want to give up nursing. Traveling will challenge you professionally, socially, psychologically, and perhaps spiritually. Some travelers need to find their niche. Once travelers experience a few assignments, they often notice how differently they feel depending on their work environment.

What is different? The work is basically the same, yet each workplace is different and has a personality of its own. For example, Susan, an experienced traveler, expresses what the right environment can do for a nurse. She finds her current assignment in Austin, Texas to be different from the places she has worked in the past. She admits that many times, she has wondered if getting into nursing was a mistake. Now, for the first time in 17 years, she actually looks forward to going to work again. She says, "The people I work with here are so much fun, and the technology is advanced enough to keep me challenged. It is like I am a new nurse starting over again. I am signing a contract with the hospital for another 18 months."

Myth 7: Traveling Is Not a Reliable Source of Income

Look at the trends in the health care industry today, and the demand in the nursing profession becomes evident. And, it is only going to increase over time.

According to a recent study published in the "Journal of the American Medical Association," the registered nurse (RN) workforce will fall 20% behind estimated requirements by the year 2020 (Ericksen, 2001).

The current employment climate for permanent nursing staff has changed over the past few years. Downsizing, layoffs, hospital closures, and mergers are creating uncertainty and employment insecurity (Smith, 1995). Dependability, adaptability, and assertiveness are more important traits to maintain employment than in the past.

If you are a nurse and are considering leaving the nursing profession, you are not alone. Nurses primarily report frustration with budget cutbacks that are affecting the quality of nursing care they can provide. On average, nurses with 5 or more years experience are leaving the field (Schaffzin, 1998) as a result.

Hospitals are merging, ordering hiring freezes, and decreasing benefits in order to cut costs to compensate for increased medical expenses. The United States spends 12% to 13% on health care, while other industrialized nations spend only 5% to 7% (Johnson, 1999). In the changing, cost-conscious environment of today, health care facilities must identify and implement strategies to promote fiscal responsibility.

Meanwhile, job security is a concept of the past. Individuals are becoming their own employers. Health care professionals can no longer rely on a single employer to promise work in return for their loyalty.

A self-employed, entrepreneurial attitude is necessary to adapt to this new environment. The good news is that work options are abundant for the self reliant, self-motivated, and proactive professional.

Kevin Lumsdon, a health care expert, explains the need for nurses to be flexible. With experience, nurses can market themselves throughout the country. They will have a hard time earning top dollar if they are bound to one community (Johnson, 1999).

According to the Bureau of Labor Statistics, employment for registered nurses is expected to grow faster than the average for all occupations through 2008, resulting in many new jobs. They attribute this fast growth to technological advances, the aging population, and experienced nurses leaving the profession.

Furthermore, the number of jobs for RNs in personnel supply services (which includes agency nursing) is projected to increase 36% by 2008. Short-term employment and on-the-job training are predicted to have the most growth.

Heath care professionals can stay ahead by being proactive trend observers. The growth potential for travel nursing is on the rise. The demand is great and will only increase as the demand for nurses increases. The demand for other health care workers will also increase as the population continues to grow and age, and the pace of technology increases.

Traveling originated in the early 1980s, when medical staffing agencies began providing their services to cover seasonal shortages in places such as Arizona, Florida, and California. Today, seasonal demand is only one of many reasons for traveling staff placement. Travel nursing is soaring as it fills in the need created by the dichotomy of cost containment versus increased demand for nurses, especially during busy seasons and high staff turnovers.

By hiring travelers, hospitals may save money and avoid having to lay off employees as needs fluctuate. Sometimes, travelers aid in the implementation of new care models by allowing permanent staff the necessary time to become educated on new procedures.

Travelers provide continuity of care when compared to local daily agency staffing. With local agency staffing, hospitals cannot be sure which local nurses will be providing coverage or if they will be available. Traveling nurses, on the other hand, are there on contract for at least 3 months. In other words, the hospital has more reliable and consistent coverage with a traveler during the time of the contract.

Experienced health care travelers have a broad knowledge base from working in so many different facilities. They can offer information about new procedures and methods that increase quality and efficiency of the workplace. Meanwhile, traveling is a tool nurses use for themselves to prevent burnout by seeking out situations where they are constantly learning and being challenged.

"Flexible staffing is in; that is a fact" (Thrailkill, 1999). The demand for health care travelers is rising as the need for nurses and other health professionals rises, and health care facilities recognize the benefits of travelers.

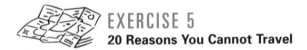

EXERCISE 5
20 Reasons You Cannot Travel

Now that you are aware of the traveling myths, take a closer look at the obstacles in your mind. Make a list of 20 reasons you cannot be a traveling health care provider. Write down 20 even if you have to include trivial reasons. For example, you may list such things as, "I have a house," "Not enough stability," or "What about my plants?"

As you read this book, keep your list in hand and see if any of your obstacles are addressed and become less of an issue as you read about being a traveler. Sometimes, just the act of writing down an obstacle makes you realize how trivial it may be.

continued

exercise 5 continued

If you still have obstacles that have not been addressed or that still feel impossible to overcome, have an idea party. Invite several friends over, and tell them what you want to do. Ask for ideas and then brainstorm. The primary way to overcome most barriers is by changing perspective. Then, take action.

If you take an assignment and you do not like it, you can decide not to travel. But if you decide not to take an assignment because you are unsure, then you will never know. Taking action of some kind is important. Action is informative. By taking action, you learn what you like and don't like. Any time you act in spite of your apprehensions, you are a success.

Taking the steps toward being a traveler may bring up any resistance you have about it. Become aware of your resistance as you read this book. Awareness can help you overcome these obstacles. Change is not easy; however, butterflies discover their wings only after they break free of their cocoons.

Reading this book is the first step toward traveling. You are gathering information. You are taking action.

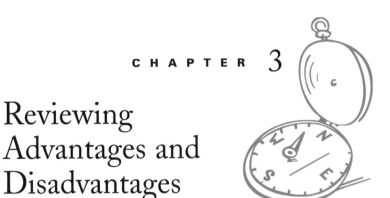

CHAPTER 3

Reviewing Advantages and Disadvantages

All decisions in life have advantages and disadvantages. Traveling is no different. You must examine your goals, priorities, and needs, because each person's situation is different. While traveling can be great for one person, it may not be for another. In this chapter, we discuss the most common advantages and disadvantages reported by travelers, examine the factors involved, and see if they apply to your situation.

THE ADVANTAGES

See the Country

Travel nursing is a great way to see the country. Basically, you can have the best of the nomadic carefree life mixed with the security of a stable life (a job and a place to live). Your basic necessities are provided for while you roam the countryside.

Living somewhere, even temporarily, can be more satisfying than vacationing there. It allows you to get to know the area's culture and intricacies that you don't have time to discover on a vacation. You acquire a more full and realistic perspective of the local culture. After all, differences in culture can exist in the same country, or even in the same town.

Knowing that you have very little time (eg, 3 months) in one place motivates you to do as much as possible. Travelers are rarely bored. They often see more of what a town has to offer in 3 months than a permanent resident does in 10 years.

Meet New People

Knowing people becomes a survival tool when you are in a strange town. It often brings out your extroverted personality. Other travelers in the area can be a great source of friendship. You can have fun swapping travel stories and suggestions. The next thing you know, you may find yourself on a big adventure with a fellow traveler you just met. Often you feel as if you have known them much longer because of your shared interest. Like you, they are new to the area, they are in the medical profession, and they want to explore.

Other travelers are easy to find. First, look around your department. If another traveler does not work in your department, ask your agency or hospital if they have other travelers staffed at or near your location.

Ask your apartment manager. Sharon found her traveling buddy on her first assignment. When she checked into her apartment, the manager at the apartment complex mentioned that he had another traveler living there. "I just went and knocked on her door," Sharon says. "We shared a bottle of wine that night and became instant friends. We took several travel assignments together. Eight years later, we are still friends. Recently, I flew to Rhode Island to attend her wedding."

Be careful. Just like anywhere else, there are some odd travelers out there, but they are usually obvious to spot. They may be avoiding personal issues or have different reasons for traveling.

Live in New and Interesting Places

Traveling puts you more in touch with your environment and the people around you. As a traveler, you have to be more aware and able to utilize your resources. It is exhilarating.

Every place is interesting in its own way. Arizona is known for its painted deserts and beautiful sunsets. Philadelphia is filled with unique character and culture. Florida has beaches. Alaska is wild, "the last frontier." Utah has a beautiful red glowing landscape. Louisiana has great Cajun food, huge trees, and scary alligators. North Carolina is friendly and full of outdoor activities such as water rafting. The Blue Ridge Drive along the Appalachian Mountains is wonderful.

Experience a Change

If you are a person who hates routine and likes change, this is the job path for you. Every 3 months, you have the opportunity to start over, literally.

You can travel at random or travel by theme. What if you set out to visit all the hot springs in the United States, see all the largest waterfalls, or snow ski at the best slopes? Or, you can simply set out to visit all your family and friends throughout the country. So many choices are available to you. You can shape your future and create your own story. Keep a journal, and you will have a memory of these unique experiences forever.

Discover Where You Want to Live

Many travelers stop traveling either because they find a place they like, or because they find a person they like. Traveling is a great way to determine where you want to live. You may travel for years, until one day the place "finds" you. One traveler, April, spent 7 years on the road before she found that special place. She took an assignment to Las Vegas, Nevada and decided to call it home. She doesn't even gamble or stay up late. What else is there to do in Vegas? Obviously, you have to live there to know the true answer to that question.

Conversely, you may have always dreamed of living in Seattle, and gathered certain ideas about it from books or movies. Traveling there allows you to try it out without making a permanent commitment. You may discover you hate rainy days.

Relocate

Perhaps you are going to relocate to a new area and are not sure where you want to work or live. Wouldn't it be great to be able to arrive at this new area with a job already lined up and a place to live? During your 3-month assignment, you can decide if you like that particular hospital and ask around about the other hospitals. You also have a chance to check out the area and decide where in town you want to live.

Earn Good Pay

Traveling not only provides you with a smooth transition from one geographical place to another, it can also help you negotiate better pay. Often, hospitals will want to hire you as permanent staff after your contract is over. Many travelers have been able to use their travel pay as leverage when discussing their pay for permanent placement.

Most of the time, you can make more money traveling than you can working in a permanent position. Some colleagues may be envious that you are doing the same job and getting paid more to do it. Do not be influenced by other people's fears. Everyone has the opportunity to travel. Many people, however, are not willing to leave the familiarity of their home, family, friends, and belongings in order to travel, even if it means more money. Remember that it is their choice to believe in the myths that keep them bound.

Susan is a traveler who used to feel bound by fear. Now she says, "Traveling is fabulous every time I get my paycheck. I make about $7 more an hour than I did at my full-time job. That does not include my housing." She explains, "I didn't travel until now because I was afraid of the unknown. I was afraid that I didn't know enough. I knew other people would use different techniques. Another traveler talked to me and resolved my fears. It is a little difficult, but not as bad as I thought."

Avoid Politics

As a traveler, you do not have to be involved in hospital politics. Your contract is between you and the staffing agency, not the hospital.

Thus, you are not as vulnerable to the changes within the hospital system. Bureaucracy will always be a factor in any work environment, but your involvement in it is a choice. You have the power to walk away and focus on your work, which is a nice advantage for your state of mind.

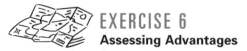

EXERCISE 6
Assessing Advantages

Think of more advantages and add them to the list. Circle the two advantages that are most important to you. Your reasons may change later, but that's okay.

- See the country.
- Meet new people.
- Live in new and interesting places.
- Discover where you want to live.
- Relocate.
- Earn good pay.
- Work in some of the finest health care facilities.
- Learn new skills and techniques.
- Avoid hospital politics.
- Experience change.
- Investigate permanent placement.
- Enhance the sense of control over your future.

It is important to be in touch with why you are traveling and what you hope to get out of it. You want to stay focused so that you don't find yourself floating around trying to remember why you started traveling in the first place. This can lead to self-doubt and inner conflict. Readdress your list every few months.

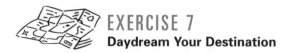

EXERCISE 7
Daydream Your Destination

Make a list of all the places you would like to go in the country and why. Then circle the top four choices and write them below. Think about it. If you take a new assignment every 3 months, you can see the top four places in 1 year of traveling.

1. _____

2. _____

3. _____

4. _____

THE DISADVANTAGES

Is the risk worth it? As Denise, an expert traveler says, "It is not all wine and roses." In this chapter, several disadvantages are presented to give you an objective view of traveling. You are the only one who knows if it is right for you. Looking at the variables of the situation will aid you in making an informed decision about the possibility of traveling.

Unsettled or No Roots

Working as a full-time traveler (going from one assignment to the next) can be unsettling. You are truly living in the moment. There is not much time to establish roots or build for the future. Your past evaporates. Will people remember you? Will you remember them? This can be great for some, but it can be uncomfortable for others. The traveling lifestyle means you rarely participate in the activities of settling down, such as developing a comfortable routine, buying a house, getting attached to the community, or acquiring material possessions.

This gypsy lifestyle requires you to adapt fast. You temporarily trade stability for adventure. Your world becomes fragmented. Some enjoy the challenges of a nomadic life. They keep in touch with friends along the way and look forward to the next adventure. Others, however, find themselves feeling empty and homesick.

You do not have to be a nomadic traveler, however. Several travelers manage to travel while enjoying home life as well. Remember that you always have the option of traveling part time. For example, Sara works as needed (PRN) in her New Jersey hometown most of the year, and travels in the winter. When she feels homesick, she returns home to her friends and family.

All types of arrangements can be worked out. Cathy is married to a farmer in Pennsylvania. Her husband loves to travel with her during his off-season. When the farming season starts again, they return home where she works at a local hospital.

You should be able to find a way to maintain a degree of certainty and stability in your life, but you still may have to sacrifice a few smaller things. Think about some things that require continual maintenance. One is growing plants. This may not seem like a big deal, but after a time their importance can grow. For example, Katie says that when she stops traveling, the first thing she is going to do is surround herself with plants and animals. Sometimes, after traveling awhile, you begin to appreciate the simple things in life, she says. On the other hand, Rose felt trapped by her possessions. After 6 years of taking care of two Belgian Sheep-dogs and maintaining a large greenhouse, she was anxious to find a way to relieve herself of her responsibilities so she could travel.

Many factors, including your family and economic situation, will determine to what degree a disadvantage will affect you. Depending on your living situation, you may need to put some of your possessions in storage. Some travelers even sell many of their possessions to free themselves from burdensome bills. Others use travel to acquire more possessions. Therefore, it is important to assess what you will really be giving up and what you will be gaining by traveling.

One traveler, Karen, uses traveling to find a place to settle down. She says, "Ultimately I am looking for a place to settle down. I don't have a home base, but I am not the normal traveler. Traveling is a vehicle to find a good place to live." Karen explains her approach in more detail. "I don't consider myself a normal traveler because I travel with two cats and a dog. I have so many things that I have to rent a moving van to go to another assignment. Finally, I usually stay in one assignment for 2 years or more before moving to the next one. This way, I maintain some stability and really give a place a chance before deciding it is not the place for me. Since I don't room with other travelers, I do feel lonely at times. I often deal with this by making sure other travelers are at the hospital during my interview. Other travelers often become like family."

One thing you cannot put in storage, though, is your family. Intimate relationships require continual maintenance. Therefore, you must really talk with your family about how long you intend to travel and what you will do to stay connected during that time. Ask each other how often you can realistically see each other during your assignment, and whether that will be enough. Can you afford the travel and long-distance calls? Make sure you take extra time while you are gone to show you are thinking of them and have not abandoned them. Some parents bring their children with them either during the summer or full time. Those who take their children often home school them. One traveler, Mike, travels with his wife and kids. While he travels, his wife advances her studies and home schools the children. They recommend The Sycamore Tree Center for Home Education. (See Appendix A.)

Makes Your Resume Look Funny

Don't worry about your resume looking unstable. Most people in health care understand the concept of traveling. The fact that you have worked in so many different facilities can be a strong point. Just make sure to indicate on your resume that these are travel assignments. This helps the interviewer avoid the misconception that you are flighty or unable to hold down a permanent job.

Be sure to note the dates and places where you work. The list will come in handy later. For example, a nurse named Olivia was called to give a deposition. She sat at one end of a long table, surrounded by lawyers, with a video camera filming her from the other end of the table. The lawyers began with questions regarding her work history. Out of the 3-hour deposition, Olivia found that her work history was the most difficult part to remember and explain.

Baffles Your Accountant

You will find that many accountants are not aware of all the tax advantages for the traveler. You have to keep yourself informed in order to get all the advantages you can out of traveling. Refer to Chapter 9 to find tax tips and resources.

Endure Several Hospital Orientations

Many facilities are moving away from requiring that you go to general hospital orientation before your department orientation. Some facilities still require the general orientation, however.

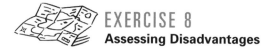

EXERCISE 8
Assessing Disadvantages

Think of any other disadvantages and add them to the list. Then circle the two disadvantages that disturb you most. Decide whether you could live with these disadvantages or not. Next, consider ways to avoid the possible disadvantages or make them work for you. Get your friends together and come up with ideas.

- Difficult to establish stability.
- Give up a degree of closeness with friends and family.
- Makes your resume look funny.
- Forget where home is.
- Want to live everywhere.
- Leave a paper trail for the mailman.
- Baffle your accountant.
- Endure several hospital orientations.
- Leave a trail of broken hearts, or have one.
- Leave belongings in storage.

It is very important to take the time now to consider the disadvantages and how to deal with them. This will determine whether you are a happy traveler. Everyone is different in how they handle the drawbacks of traveling. Many travelers have creative ways to deal with these disadvantages. Overall, you have to assess your values and what you want at this stage in your life.

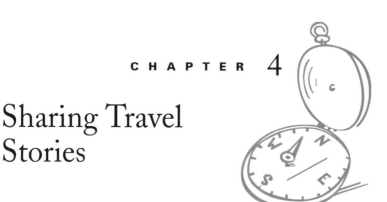

CHAPTER 4

Sharing Travel Stories

Even after reading the advantages and disadvantages of traveling, and applying them to your life, would you still like to hear the real story directly from "the horse's mouth"? Maybe you have questioned a few travelers at your workplace, but wondered if they were accurate. Here are the inside views of experienced travelers from all over the country, describing their true feelings about what it's like to be a traveler. To provide an objective portrayal of traveling, a special effort has been made to include optimistic and pessimistic viewpoints from travelers.

QUOTES FROM EXPERIENCED TRAVELERS

Traveling is "a diamond one day and a stone the next."
By Charlotte Culpepper, RN

The main reason I started traveling in 1989 was because I wanted to go to California, to cope with the empty nest syndrome. I took an assignment in San Jose. The first week I was there, my car was stolen. I drove a rental car the entire assignment.

Then the earthquake came (7.5 on the Richter scale). I was in my apartment. Everything began to shake. All the lights went out and the phone went dead. I tried to remember what you were supposed to do during an earthquake, and ended up just sitting there in the dark. It didn't really disturb me until later, when I saw all the people who were killed during the earthquake. But I have no regrets. I fell in love with San Francisco and am still traveling.

"Traveling is enlightening."
By Patricia Tubin, RN

Traveling opens up a whole new world. It is great for me because I am not married and my children are all grown. I was a little naive on my first assignment. When they said I would have a furnished apartment, I thought that would include a TV and appliances. If I had known, I would have brought much more than I did.

Traveling is "educational."
By Penny Nichols, CST

You learn a lot about different areas of the country. I started traveling because I was 30 years old and had never been out of Houston, Texas. I would say that I am more independent now than I was before I started traveling. I had 6 1/2 years of experience before I started traveling. I have learned how to cut down on my packing. I would recommend a laptop computer to keep in touch with the rest of the world. I do my banking online, and my mail goes to my mom. She sends me any of the important stuff. It's funny: when you travel, the trees are all different. In Mississippi, it's oak trees, Louisiana is cypress trees, and Alaska is pine trees.

In Alaska, it was moose and bear, and in Louisiana, it was snakes and alligators. I took a swamp tour in Louisiana. There were five or six alligators surrounding the boat. I even fed one.

Traveling is "flexibility."
By Tony Trusty II, CST

I have been traveling for 3 years now. Originally, I traveled to escape the politics of the workplace. Now I continue to travel for the change.

I like to keep moving. My life is different now than before I started traveling. Traveling has forced me to be organized. I also used to be quiet and sort of shy. Now, I don't have any trouble talking to people. You have to get out and talk to people when you are traveling.

I have stayed with one company for most of my assignments so I have retirement investing and other benefits. When I first started traveling, I would just take whatever came to me because I didn't know what to look for. Now I ask a lot of questions before I take the assignment and prevent myself from being abused in the workplace. I get them to tell me what kind of caseload I can expect, if I will be expected to change services frequently, and the pay.

Traveling is "negotiable."
By Denise Calhoun, CRNA

My first travel assignment could very well have been my last. The housing accommodations were provided in the hospital in a ward that had been closed. The beds were so uncomfortable that I became sleep deprived. The meals in the cafeteria were free, but the food was inedible. The staff did not welcome travelers, and the convenience of having a pool of 18 traveling nurses in-house was often abused.

We became notorious for having extravagant parties in our hospital suites. Although our in-house, off-duty behavior was called into question, the quality of our professional performance was impeccable.

I learned that all assignments will have faults and the outcome would depend on my attitude. I came away from that assignment with 18 of the dearest friends of my life, a beautiful figure from the weight loss, and debt-free from the overtime. But, most of all, I gained insight about the travel nursing industry and the benefit of negotiating contracts.

It is best to be remembered for the quality of your work. The staff will scrutinize your work and their recommendations may often influence whether you are offered an extension on your contract. Maintaining a good rapport keeps the door open and allows you to negotiate the next contract. It is a good idea to maintain a current resume with letters of reference from each assignment.

After that first assignment, I traveled for 13 years. As time went by, I focused on career development and chose assignments that were beneficial to me. I found that everything was negotiable and my credentials were my bargaining chips.

Traveling is "an adventure."
By Margaret Washburn, RN

I have been traveling for 8 years. It was a big change, but you have to bite off a little bit at a time. My sister said she would take care of my dog. I sold my house and two cars, and put a few things in storage and kept the rest. My suggestion on your first assignment is to go someplace where you know either a friend or relative.

I also highly recommend international travel. It really opens your eyes. "Man cannot discover new oceans unless he has the courage to lose sight of the shore." This is an anonymous quote that reminds me of traveling because it does take a lot of courage. And remember, you can always go back to where you were.

Traveling is "the only way to go."
By Paul Baker, RN

Travelers get trashed. Since you are getting paid a lot of money, you cannot sit for 5 minutes. I always get assigned to the sickest patients and the most difficult surgeons. Hospitals that use travelers are usually the worst conditions to work. One place I went to in Miami was a dive. The next place never oriented me. I didn't even know where to find any supplies.

By being thrown into situations, however, I have plenty of experience. I can do any surgical case that comes my way. Traveling is the only way to go because nurses do not make enough money for what they do. You must travel to survive.

Traveling is "exciting."
By Kim Groves, CST

My first assignment to Michigan was exciting. I went to a place I had never even heard of before. The people were great. I met up with two people whose families were multimillionaires. We went boating every day after work.

You never know what you are going to get. You may end up working at a place with the latest technology, or you may end up working in the backwoods, wondering if they have even read any medical journals. Traveling is rewarding, though, because you know you have the ability to work at any facility.

It is also appealing because you are out of the hospital politics. Once you walk through the door, the countdown begins. You know you will only be there for 3 months.

Traveling is " fun."
By Brian Salensky, CST

Traveling is fun because you get to see everything and you don't have to pay for it yourself. The only disadvantage is that often you are sent to areas that have low staffing. I have known travelers that have had bad experiences, but most of those had to do with personality conflicts.

Traveling is "a great experience."
By Chris Ransom, CST

Traveling is a great experience, but you have to be self-reliant. My new approach is to find two large companies that have several assignment locations and one small company that pays more. That way, I can change companies depending on what my needs are at the time.

I feel so much more in control of my life since I started traveling. I have plenty of money. In December, I am going to take the entire month off and visit my family.

Traveling is "freeing."
By Pam Mularcik, RN

Travel nursing appeals to the gypsy in me. It feeds my independence. I am a free spirit and I like to try different things and meet different people. To be a good traveling nurse, you have to be a people person, flexible, and know what to do to come into a new situation and be part of the group.

You have to go with the flow. I also try to make the same amount of money or more each time that I travel. I think everyone should try traveling if they can.

WHAT IT ALL SAYS

Life is a series of experiences. Traveling is like pushing the accelerator on life. It gives you the opportunity to experience more than many people do in a lifetime. Even if a person tries traveling and decides it is not for them, they rarely regret the experience.

One traveler, Beth, went to Alaska for the summer. She arrived just after the hospital had finished a nursing strike. The nurses were still bitter toward travelers and working there was difficult. Beth really liked outdoor activities, but did not like worrying about the bears and moose on her hikes. Needless to say, she could not wait to leave Alaska. If given the opportunity, however, she would do it all again. The experience was invaluable. She learned more about herself and about another piece of the world.

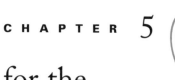

CHAPTER 5

Preparing for the Application Process

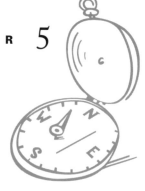

Now that you have read the actual accounts of travelers, do you want to be one yourself? If so, this is a must-read chapter. It will inform you about the preparation required to travel, so that you will be one step ahead of the game. Not only does being prepared portray professionalism, it also may help you land that ultimate assignment. An agency cannot submit you to a hospital until your file is complete. If you are not prepared, the assignment may go to someone else. Don't let this happen to you! If you already know you want to travel, get your paperwork together before contacting the agencies. Most agencies require the same information and documentation.

ASSESS YOUR READINESS

Before applying with an agency, it is a good idea first to assess your readiness. Most agencies require you to have at least 1 year of experience in your desired specialty. If you have been a nurse for 15 years, but only have 6 months of labor and delivery experience, do not expect to work in labor and delivery when you travel. Get the experience now to prepare you for the type of travel assignment you want later.

The medical profession is not known for planning ahead. Granted, needs fluctuate rapidly in medicine. One of the first questions that the agency or the hospital will ask is: When are you available to travel?

Usually, the sooner you can travel, the better. Most facilities understand that you will need time to give 2-weeks' notice, obtain your temporary nursing license, and drive to the assignment. If the facility uses travelers often and has a constant need, they may be willing to plan a future starting date. Otherwise, they may want you right away.

WHAT YOU NEED TO GET STARTED

If you don't know what to expect when applying for an agency, you may find yourself overwhelmed at the amount of paperwork and documentation involved. The information below can be used as a general guide so you can start preparing for the process.

If you know you want to travel, complete your paperwork *before* you call the agencies. This will make the process go much smoother, and will show that you are both prepared and professional. Keep copies of all your documents in a safe place.

Build a portfolio. When you apply with another agency, you can simply pull out your folder and fax the copies. One nurse scans all her documents in the computer, and then e-mails them to the agencies.

Keep these documents with you at all times when you travel. Invariably, something gets lost and you will be asked to send another copy. All the documents listed on page 30 have to be accounted for before you can work.

Making your own generic forms can save time. When applying with several agencies, the paperwork can become very repetitive and labor intensive. If you do not have a computer to make generic copies, use a copy machine.

You can change company forms into generic application forms by covering the company name and logo with correction fluid or tape, or cutting out the company identification. You can then use these to apply to other companies. Some companies won't accept generic forms, but some will. A typed resume is generally accepted instead of the application form, or at least in place of the work history section of the form. If attaching resumes or generic forms, write "SEE ATTACHED" in corresponding lines of the agency's form.

It is not the staffing agency you need to impress, but the hospital. The agency is happy to have a skilled person to place. But be warned! Do not have more than one agency market you to the same facility. This makes you look unprofessional both to the agencies and the hospital.

Unfortunately, traveling requires more paperwork all the time. Regulating agencies have added routine tests for nurses. The agency and the hospital must have evidence that you have read material on fire safety, electrical safety, proper body mechanics, age competencies, and more. These tests will be administered to you at some point, either by the agencies or by the hospital. Sometimes you will also be tested on your knowledge of medications.

Forms

To get started, you need forms from the agency, such as their application form and a skills checklist. You can originate many of the other documents yourself. You need to provide the agency with copies of your resume and your medical history, usually including a tuberculosis (TB) skin test (purified protein derivative, or PPD; no more than 1 year old) or chest x-ray (within the last 2 years), annual physical, and immunization record. Personal documentation including copies of your social security card, driver's license, nursing license, passport for international travel, current basic cardiac life support (BCLS, front and back) certification, and any additional certifications required for your specialty area also need to be submitted.

References

Find two professional associates you have worked with who respect your work and are willing to act as references. Make sure they do not mind getting occasional letters and calls for references. Most agencies require two written references. Many of them prefer to get the reference directly from the source, and will not accept a written reference that you send in. Make sure to ask how they prefer to receive the letter of reference.

Skills Checklist

The skills checklist form is probably the most time consuming to complete. The agency provides its own checklist for you to rate yourself and your own abilities. This list is used by the facility to see if you will meet their needs. Even though you want to impress the facility, do not exaggerate your proficiency. This could result in uncomfortable situations. You are not expected to know everything. The institution does not expect to teach short-term health care professionals. Therefore, they often try to place you according to your current level of skill and experience.

You can also use the checklist to your benefit. You have the option of claiming ignorance on duties or procedures you abhor.

Do not be intimidated by the skills checklist. Several items on the list may be unfamiliar. You may feel like you are trying to read a foreign language. This is normal. Remember, you are not required to know everything. Different parts of the country and different facilities use different terminology, procedures, and equipment.

Medical History

As mentioned earlier, the PPD skin test must be less than 1 year old. Alaska is the exception, however. Alaskan facilities usually require a TB skin test to be no more than 3 months old. If you have been tested at work within the last year, you can go to the employee health nurse and ask her for a copy of the results on company letterhead for your records.

If you have not been tested within the past year, the employee health nurse will be happy you brought it to her attention. You can request a test and a copy of the results.

The physical is basically a statement by a physician that you are healthy enough to work. This should be simple to obtain from one of the doctors with whom you work.

Make a copy of your immunizations. New regulations require your measles, mumps, and rubella (MMR) to be no more than 10 years old. Some agencies are enforcing this new regulation and some are not, so make sure to ask. You also need proof of your varicella immunization and hepatitis B series. If you can't find your hepatitis B series, you can simply write down that you would like to decline on receiving the hepatitis B series at this time and sign it. If you truly have not had your hepatitis B series of shots, it is advised, but not mandatory.

Professional Certifications and Experience

If you are a nurse, you need to send a copy of your current nursing license from your home state. To save time and effort, you can take a short cut by failing to mention your other active licenses until a time when they are more relevant. Otherwise, be prepared to send copies and note all the license numbers you have on the application form.

DOCUMENT CHECKLIST (COPIES)

☐ PPD (less than 1 year old)
☐ Annual physical
☐ Immunization record (documentation/titre)
☐ Current nursing license
☐ BCLS (front and back)
☐ Social Security card
☐ Driver's license
☐ Professional certifications
☐ Two references
☐ Application to the agency
☐ Resume (optional)
☐ Skills checklist
☐ Hepatitis B series or declination

Applying for Licensure

If you are a licensed professional, you need to obtain a license in the state where you will be working. The agency usually has the information you need on how long it will take to obtain your license.

All the state nursing boards have different rules and requirements. A few require you to have Continuing Education Units (CEU) in particular subjects, such as AIDS or child abuse. Some nursing boards take a long time to process paperwork, while others do not. You may be able to obtain a temporary license, which allows you to get your license sooner, but it expires in a few months.

When you talk to the nursing board, note the name of the person you are speaking with to establish a contact person. Find out if that state will issue you a temporary license. Temporary licenses allow you to work in a particular state anywhere from 1 to 6 months, depending on the state.

It is recommended that you apply for a permanent license at the same time you apply for the temporary one. You may decide you want to extend your assignment or take another assignment in the same state. When you finish an assignment, contact the board and have them file your license as inactive. An inactive license is still on file, but you do not have to pay the renewal fees each year unless you reactivate the license.

The time required to get your license is an important factor to consider. Some states are referred to as "walk-through states." A walk-through state has a nursing board that allows you to walk in with all the required paperwork and get a temporary license the same day.

Even if you are going to a walk-through state, it is still a good idea to send in the paperwork before you leave, to allow extra time for processing. Sometimes you will be required to get notarized copies of your current license, fingerprints, and passport photos.

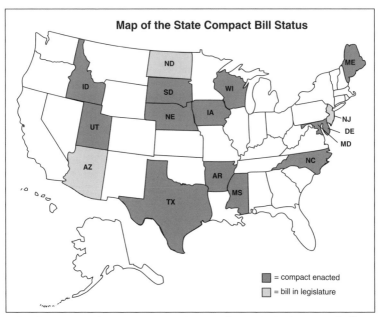

FIGURE 5-1. Map of state compact bill status. The dark-shaded states indicate compact enacted and the light-shaded states have a bill in legislature as of March 2001. See the NCSBN web site, www.ncsbn.org, for the latest compact update. (Reprinted by permission of the National Council of State Boards of Nursing, Inc. Chicago, IL. From the NCSBN Web site www.ncsbn.org.)

Make sure you know where the nursing board is located so you can allot enough time to drive to the board a day or two before your assignment. If the state is not a walk-through state, ask them how long it takes to obtain a temporary nursing license. In some states, it can take up to 8 weeks.

Just recently, new legislation called the Nurse Licensure Compact was passed that eliminates the need to apply for licensure in some states. According to *HT Magazine* (2001), several states currently are involved in this legislation: Arkansas, Delaware, Iowa, Maine, Maryland, North Carolina, Texas, Utah, and Wisconsin. These states are known as "compact states," because they recognize each other's nursing licenses as they would a driver's license. If you are a permanent resident in any of the compact states, you can work in any other compact state without having to apply for a new license.

The goal is for nurses to have privileges nationwide. This is very great news for travelers. For more detailed information and updates, log onto www.ncsbn.org.

If you want to work in a particular state, for instance, Florida or California, be certain to find out what their licensing requirements are before contracting with the agency. This will give you time to prepare in case the agency has an immediate assignment.

All this preparation may seem overwhelming; however, if you break it down you can control the pace. Being prepared makes the process much easier and makes you appear more experienced and professional. Before you know it, you are ready to travel. Take it step by step. Have fun!

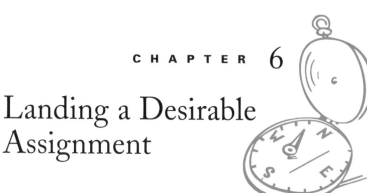

CHAPTER 6

Landing a Desirable Assignment

Paperwork is only one aspect of being prepared for travel. Your mental preparation also makes a big difference. You need to be clear about what you want in order to select a good agency. This chapter explains the step-by-step process of finding the best agency and assignment for you. Not only will you understand the process better, but you will also know the important questions to ask at appropriate times so that you can make more informed decisions. First, let's begin with the questions you should ask yourself before looking for an agency.

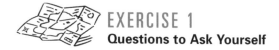

EXERCISE 1
Questions to Ask Yourself

Ask yourself these questions before taking the first step.

1. Does my personality fit that of a typical traveler?
2. What is the main reason I want to travel?
3. Do I have all my documentation ready?
4. Can I travel within a month or sooner, if asked?
5. Where do I want to go? Why?
6. What is the most important quality I am looking for in an agency? Rank the following in order of importance:
   a. High pay
   b. Friendliness
   c. Organization
   d. Housing meets my preference (shared or private)
   e. Professionalism
   f. Well-established institution
   g. Desirable location

continued

exercise 1 continued

h. Has many assignment locations
i. Good long term incentives
j. Health insurance effective immediately
k. Tax advantage programs
l. Staff my unique specialty area

Once you have addressed these questions, review your answers. Use the information to guide you in choosing an agency that is the right "fit" for you and your goals.

RESEARCH THE AGENCIES

Much of the research has already been done for you in this book. Lists of agencies and resources are provided for you in the back of this book. You can use this information as a guide. For additional information, you can look at each agency's web site.

Joining the Association of Traveling Nurses (at www.travelnursingcentral.com) is also a way to obtain additional information and guidance. As a member, you have access to their brokerage services, agency rankings, expert advice, newsletters, annual conventions, and more. The brokerage service can do the research for you to find the agency that best matches your desires. They also use ongoing nursing surveys to rank agencies according to nursing satisfaction, so you know what to expect from the agency.

Furthermore, they help you minimize your paperwork by keeping your file in their database and informing you when you need to update it. Later, when you want to apply to an agency, all you have to do is call them and ask them to fax over your file.

CALL THE AGENCIES

Once you decide you have enough information to work with, narrow your selection to the top six agencies that appeal to you most, based on your previously assessed goals, and start calling these companies. Talking to them on the phone helps you get a feel for what they are about and how they treat their travelers. Then, after talking to them, narrow your choices further to three or four agencies.

Many travelers sign up with several agencies at the same time. Signing up with more than one agency allows you to have more choices in benefits and places to go. Make sure that only one agency actually submits your resume to the hospital, however. The hospital wants to identify you with one agency.

Most agencies have developed incentives to persuade you to work exclusively for them. You can earn paid vacations, free continuing education units, bonuses, and investments in 401(k) plans by staying with one agency. On the other hand, if you choose to work with more than one agency, you may have more freedom, choices, and negotiation power. Once again, being clear on your goals and intentions is really important here. You must weigh the options and choose which approach works best for you.

After traveling 7 years, Sheila shares her approach to agencies. First, she sets criteria for herself on how much money she will work for and what "perks" she requires. She then calls several agencies to see who will meet those criteria. She likes to work with the smaller agencies because they take more time with her concerns and work with her one on one. She also feels that negotiations are easier with smaller agencies.

TAKE GOSSIP WITH A GRAIN OF SALT

"What is the best agency?" is always the big question among travelers. The answer is that the best agency is the one that works for you. Although agencies offer similar competitive packages, they have very different characteristics such as location, length of time in business, specialties staffed, and benefits offered.

Once you have gathered information on those unique characteristics and matched them to your goals, you can find a fit for you. For example, if your goal is to travel out of the country, you may want to sign up with an agency that staffs internationally. If you are looking for a more professional agency, you may want to sign up with an agency that is staffed by all RN's or has a management approach. If your goal is to maintain as much stability as possible while traveling, find an agency with the best long-term benefits and stay with them.

Every agency is unique and has value for the traveler. You may find that although one traveler had a bad experience with an agency, that same company may work great for you. On the other hand, you may talk to one person who loves an agency, and then have a terrible experience with that agency yourself.

One traveler, Robert, summed it up when he said, "People have had good and bad experiences with all the companies. The key is to find a company you like, or better yet, a recruiter you trust."

PERSONAL RECRUITER

When you call the agency, you are assigned a personal recruiter. Remember to write down the name of your recruiter. If you cannot remember your recruiter's name, however, it's okay. The agency operator should have the name of your recruiter on file.

Recruiters can make or break your travel experience, especially if it is your first time. They become your connection to the rest of your future world. Develop a relationship with them. One traveler, Rick, describes the relationship with the recruiter as "feeling like you are in orbit and the recruiter is your lifeline. If there isn't two-way communication, you feel like someone has cut the tether and you're floating out in space."

When you are negotiating with the agency, remember that *you* are making money for *them*. If you do not work, they do not make money. Have a place in mind you want to go, but try to be flexible. Agencies usually have a wide selection. For example, if you want, you can call several agencies and ask if they have any openings in Santa Barbara, California.

If you don't have a place in mind, just call and ask the agencies what good assignments they have. They will tell you all sorts of appetizing things. They are not called recruiters for nothing. When an assignment sounds interesting to you, request more details. Often the recruiter has information about the size of the hospital, the requested start date, and the amount of pay offered.

SHARING INFORMATION

The recruiter then sends you a packet that contains information about the company, an application form, and a skills checklist. Most companies now have their own web sites. Many travelers are being referred to web sites where they can apply online. If you do not use or do not have access to online submission, you can fax your paperwork to the agency. Once you give the recruiter permission, he or she faxes your credentials to the hospital. Next, you will be called for an interview.

THE INTERVIEW

Usually, the institution contacts you soon after they receive your paperwork. Typically, the supervisor for the department calls to interview you on the phone. The supervisor may ask you a few questions about your skills and experience. Then he or she asks if you have any questions.

You need to be ready with a few questions of your own. Remember, the interview is a two-way process. The hospital is interviewing you. Meanwhile, you are evaluating the hospital as well as the agency. It is important to find out if the department is familiar with travelers, what shift they are trying to fill, how large the department is, and the nurse-to-patient ratio.

The interview process usually doesn't take very long, but it is important to get your questions answered, too. The interviewer already knows an opening is available and that you are experienced. Therefore, the supervisor may offer you the position at the time of the interview.

You can say that you need time to think about it, but keep in mind that it's more than likely you are not the only one applying for this position. If they talk to another traveler who commits right away, then you may miss out on the opportunity.

Some positions fill before you can even get your paperwork to them. One time a nurse was interested in an 8-week assignment on an island in Alaska. The opening was filled before she could think about getting the paperwork in. It all depends on the demand for the area you are applying for.

If you decide to accept the position, spend time asking more detailed questions about the assignment. The assignment may contain hidden expenses or inconveniences. For example, one nurse, Jason, who worked in Philadelphia, found that travelers were not allowed to park at the hospital. Another traveler, Paige, reported heavy construction at one of her assignments, where she had to park a mile away and walk the rest of the way into work.

Questions to Ask the Institution
1. What shift are you trying to fill?
2. Do you currently have any travelers staffed?
3. Do you usually have an ongoing need for travelers?
4. What is the size of the hospital and the department?
5. What is the nurse-to-patient ratio?
6. How is the parking at the hospital?
7. How soon do you need someone?
8. Why are you in need of staff at this time?
9. What is your float policy?
10. How much overtime can I anticipate?

ACCEPTING THE ASSIGNMENT

Your acceptance of an assignment is initially a verbal commitment. You can make this commitment directly with the hospital, or wait and tell your recruiter.

Most assignment contracts are for 13 weeks (or 3 months), but you can find assignments for as little as 4 to 8 weeks. Many assignments have an ongoing need. While on assignment, you will often be asked if you would like to extend your time there. If you want to stay in an area, you can usually extend your contract every 3 months for up to a year. One year is often the informal maximum time allotted for a traveler to extend. After a year, the institution usually feels you should make a decision to become permanent or travel elsewhere.

SIGNING THE CONTRACT

The next step is to put your verbal commitment in writing. This is also when the agency puts their commitments to you in writing.

Whatever you do, always make sure you have a signed contract between you and the agency before traveling. Never take an assignment without negotiating your benefits. Be cautious if the agency does not have a contract.

If they do not have a contract document for you to sign, draft one on your own and have them sign it. You need to clearly understand the agreements before you leave to work in another state, and especially another country. Not having a contract is bad business.

The contract should include (at minimum):
1. Where you are going to work (location and specialty)
2. The start and finish dates of your assignment
3. What your pay will be, including overtime pay, bonuses, travel reimbursement
4. How many hours you are guaranteed
5. What benefits you will receive
6. Whether you are expected to float
7. What your housing situation will be (private or shared)

Make sure to keep a copy of the final contract. A contract should guarantee you 36 to 40 hours a week. The hospital guarantees your agency those hours. You need to know that if their census is low, the hospital is not going to send you home without pay.

You are not committed until you have signed the contract (Fig. 6-1). Don't sign until you are comfortable with the agency, the hospital, and the contract. Take your time, and keep your current job until you have made your final decision. After deciding, give your 2-weeks' notice, and then join the world of traveling.

SAMPLE CONTRACT

We want to thank you for taking the this assignment with Travel Nurse International and welcome you to the world of Rapid Response. We hope that your experience will be personally and professionally rewarding. Rapid Response assignments are different than Standard Travel assignments. You are paid more per hour so that you can respond quickly, be flexible and work with the fact that your travel, housing and assignments are arranged in a short amount of time. Below are some facts you need to know.

1. You will be paid $____ per hour to work in the _____ Unit for____ weeks at _____ with overtime being paid according to the laws of the state you are working in. Your shift will be determined by the hospital. Your pay week is set by the hospital or may start the first day you work. You need to carefully and clearly fill out the enclosed sign-in sheet. Please make sure you have your supervisor sign off for each day you work. Time sheets are to be faxed to _____ within 12 hours of your work week. Failure to do so will result in a one-week delay in your paycheck.
2. Orientation Information
   Start Date:_____ Time:_____Location:_____.
   Contact:_____Hospital Address:_____.
   Dress Code: Uniforms/Scrubs provided? Yes/No
   Special Information: If you are orienting in your unit on the first day of your assignment, you may be required to complete an additional general Hospital *Orientation.* Your supervisor will notify you if a subsequent hospital orientation is required.
3. You might be asked to float to another unit or work a different shift. As Rapid Responders, this is an expectation based upon qualifications and client policy and needs.
4. If you drive to your assignment you will be reimbursed at $____ per mile (maximum of $____ each way) from your home to the city where your hospital is located. We will include this payment in your first check, if you make a note of the miles on your first time sheet. You will not be paid for miles you drive from your accommodations to the hospital. You are responsible for your own transportation to and from the hospital each day unless otherwise determined by TNI. Transportation, when provided by TNI, will be at the sole discretion of TNI. Misuse of the privilege may result in your being personally responsible for transportation or in termination of your assignment, in which case item #6 becomes applicable.
5. We provide housing for you (including basic utilities). Housing arrangments/ assignments are at the sole discretion of TNI. Depending on the length of your assignment you may be housed in hotels, rental apartments, or houses.

FIGURE 6-1. Sample agency contract. (Reprinted with permission from Travel Nurse International). *(continued)*

Housing is double occupancy and, in most cases, one person per room in a hotel, apartment, or house. You are responsible for your own telephone and cable, and their appropriate deposits, when staying a rental unit. When staying in a hotel, TNI pays for room and taxes, while you pay for telephone, incidentals, etc. You may be placed in a hotel room first until other accommodations are available. If you smoke and have a roommate, you will be asked to smoke outside. Pets are not allowed on Rapid Response assignments. Occasionally, on some Rapid Response assignments you will receive a $_____/ day (non-taxable) housing allowance, and you will be responsible for you transportation and mileage to and from work. In addition, when under this option you are required to notify the hospital, your TNI recruiter and the housing department of your address and phone number before starting orientation.

6. If you are traveled and housed at an assignment to which you have committed, and you fail to honor your contract with TNI, all travel, housing and deposit expenses paid by TNI will be deducted from any money still owned you. You will be billed for any remaining balance on housing, travel and licensing and/or deposit expense incurred by TNI on your behalf in the case of any such breach in contract.

7. You are being contracted to work an average of_____ hours per week and may be scheduled to work additional hours. Please let us know if you are not scheduled for these hours, keeping in mind that most Rapid Response contracts do not have guarantees.

8. Complete the enclosed I-9 and W-4 form, and fax to _____. Travel and housing will not be provided until we receive your signed contract, W-4 and I-9. Please sign below that you have read this letter and fax everything to TNI immediately at _____.

My signature indicates my willingness to comply with this letter of understanding.

_____   _____
Nurse   Date   TNI   Date

FIGURE 6-1. (Continued) Sample agency contract. (Reprinted with permission from Travel Nurse International).

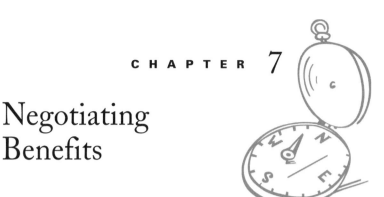

CHAPTER 7

Negotiating Benefits

Health care travel can be lucrative, especially if you know what to expect. Make sure you know what you are getting before you go through all the preparation and agency research. This chapter discusses the differences between standard and above average financial benefits, provides information about benefits that are negotiable, and explains long-term incentives.

THE STANDARD PACKAGE

The standard package should include pay, health insurance, housing, travel to and from your assignment, and a guaranteed number of hours. If any of the aforementioned is missing, then move on to another agency. In a standard package, look for the following.

Pay

While the national mean salary of a staff RN is $44,450 or $21.37 per hour, the hourly rate for a registry nurse is slightly higher than the rate for similar staff nurses in your area. This is because they do not receive benefits, which can represent 30% to 50% of a staff RN's salary (Willard, 2000). The pay for a traveling nurse ranges from $17 to $33 per hour plus free housing. Different specialties pay differently.

Pay is dependent on your location rather than on your experience level. Completion bonuses are commonly offered, or can be negotiated.

Health Insurance

Yes, travel companies provide health insurance. A few travel companies have insurance that is effective immediately. Regardless, make sure to inquire about the coverage. The fast plans sometimes are limited in coverage when compared to other plans.

Many companies have insurance that is effective approximately 30 days (1 month) after you have been on assignment. Notice the word "approximately." Sometimes the insurance does not activate until the first of the month. For example, if you start an assignment on September 12, you might think the insurance is effective on October 12, right? It may not be effective until after the first of the *next* month (November 1). If you had started the assignment on September 1, however, then the insurance would be effective on October 1—the first of a month. Be sure to ask whether "a month" actually means 1 month.

Independent insurance is another option. It allows you to avoid waiting 30 days for your insurance to be effective each time you switch companies. Often your car insurance agent will also be able to find you health insurance. You can also search the Internet by logging onto www.quotesmith.com or www.Healthaxis.com.

When searching for an independent insurance company, make sure to ask if they cover preventive care, lab testing, and previous conditions. One affordable insurance company is Unicare. Unicare insurance is provided only to those living in one of the following states, however: California, Texas, Georgia, Illinois, Indiana, and Virginia.

Another option is USAA (www.usaa.com). USAA is a company used mostly by military personnel, but their services are also available to civilians. In addition to insurance, they offer mail and banking services for people who travel.

When you are in between assignments, you also have the option of going on what is called "COBRA" (which is short for Consolidated Omnibus Budget Reconciliation Act, the federal law that allows temporary continuation of health benefits). This means you can pay a monthly fee to continue with the insurance from your last company. The agencies are required to allow you to keep this COBRA insurance for up to 18 months after your assignment if you are not covered by another insurance company.

One nurse says her COBRA insurance costs her $144 a month. She figures it's better than the independent insurance she had been keeping, because it is a group policy. The price is only slightly more than what she paid for her independent insurance. To keep this COBRA insurance policy going, she plans on taking an assignment with this same company once every 18 months.

The staffing agency will reimburse you a preset amount to cover your independent health insurance. The amount they give you per month is usually more than enough to cover the cost of your insurance.

Rent-Free Housing

Rent-free housing is a nice benefit, especially if you are not paying for a house elsewhere. The money you earn accumulates much faster. Think about it: otherwise, the majority of a person's paycheck goes to rent or mortgage payments.

The housing coordinator will find you an apartment in the area. Keep in mind that the housing coordinators have not seen your apartment with their own eyes. They rely on word of mouth and advertising. For the most part, they usually do a good job of finding a place and are careful about keeping you out of bad areas of town.

When you call to find out your new address, ask what is included in the apartment. If you really want a television or a washer and dryer, request them. Also, ask how close the apartments are located to the hospital. Usually you will be placed in an apartment, but one traveler reported an assignment in which she was placed in a nice house across the street from the hospital. You never know what to expect. One traveler, Tom, said he was placed in a cabin near the hospital in Colorado.

Once you find out the name and location of the apartment, you can do your own investigative work. Most apartments have web sites now. You can also call the hospital and ask them if they know anything about the apartments. Check with apartment locator services or realtors in the area for additional information.

The housing must meet your standards. Usually the housing is nice because the agencies want their travelers to be happy. If you get to your apartment and discover you don't like it, you can refuse to stay there.

The agency will find you a new place. One traveler, Diana, did not like her apartment. She checked into a hotel room until they found her adequate housing. She then sent them the bill for the hotel.

Some agencies provide free private housing, and some require shared housing. Enough agencies provide private housing that you should not have to share housing.

Shared housing can have its advantages, however. With shared housing, you may have a "buddy" to explore with in your new location. On the other hand, sharing could be a nightmare. Ask the housing agent to tell you a little about your roommate ahead of time. The housing agent will match you up with a roommate of the same gender and smoking preference.

Sometimes, you may be lucky enough not to have another traveler assigned to live with you. In that case, you may find yourself in a two-bedroom apartment, all to yourself, for free. This gives your family and friends a place sleep if they visit.

Do not let an agency put you in a two-bedroom apartment because they require shared housing, and then ask you to pay the difference when another traveler is not assigned to your place. This happened to a new traveler who did not know any better. The reason a traveler may not be assigned to you could be that your genders or smoking preferences are different, or simply that no more travelers took an assignment with your agency at that hospital at that time. This is not your fault. You should not have to pay for a two-bedroom apartment, if you end up lucky enough to be alone in one.

Some agencies are starting to require you to pay a deposit on your apartment, while other agencies pay the deposit for you. The deposit is refundable at the end of the assignment, if the apartment is left in good shape.

Usually, the agency will allow you to arrive at your apartment 48 hours before your actual start date at the hospital. If the apartment is ready and you want to show up earlier, you should be able to negotiate extra days for a small fee.

You also have the option of finding your own apartment and letting the company reimburse you. The company pays you a set amount based on the cost of living for the area. No matter how much your apartment cost, the company will pay you the same amount. In other words, if the company decides to pay you $700 a month for housing, and you find an apartment for $500, you can pocket the $200. Smart shoppers can come out ahead. Many travelers investigate apartments online. One web site address is www.allapartments.com.

Regardless of who picks the apartment, locating your housing is the beginning of your wild experiences as a traveler. You find yourself driving in an area you have never been before, and yet there is a home waiting for you. Either way, it is like a treasure hunt.

Questions to Ask the Housing Agent

1. Name, location, and contact information for apartment manager
2. How close is the apartment to the hospital?
3. Are a washer and a dryer inside?
4. Will I have my own private bath (in shared housing)?
5. What amenities does the complex have?
6. What do you furnish in the apartment besides furniture (microwave, TV)?
7. What utilities are paid for, and what will I need to hook up ahead of time?
8. What size beds are furnished?
9. What can you tell me about my roommate (shared housing)?
10. What can you tell me about the crime rate in the area?
11. How many other travelers are residing in the complex?
12. Any other potential cost involved with the housing?
13. How soon can I move in, and what is the expected move-out date?

Travel Reimbursement

The staffing agencies will pay you a certain amount per mile for travel to and from your destination. Most of them have a maximum limit to how much they will pay, based on the distance you need to travel. For example, they might say, "We will pay you 20 cents per mile up to $400 each way." After you have spent $400, you are on your own money. Unless you are an extravagant spender, the allotted amount is usually more than enough to get to your destination. You should not end up paying more than $200 extra to get anywhere, if you pay anything at all.

Whatever money you do not use, you can keep. Some travelers camp along the way. They have a blast, and save money at the same time.

Usually, you will drive to your assignment. If the assignment requires that you fly, however, you may be offered rental car allowance as well. Car rental is considered taxable income at the end of the year unless you send the receipts for your car to the agency. Once the agency has your receipts, they can prove that you used the money for a rental car and won't have to deduct taxes from it. Make sure you fax them copies of your receipts.

The hospitals are usually more than happy to let you use their fax machine to communicate with your agency. If you do not decide to get a rental car or you find a cheaper one, the agency will still send you the same amount of money for your rental. You can do anything you want with the money you did not spend on car rental.

Before you agree to accept a rental car allowance from the agency, check on the rates in the area. For example, one traveler went to Alaska with a $500 a month rental car allowance. She thought this would be plenty. When she got there, she discovered that the rental car rates in Alaska were $700 to $1000 a month. If she had known this, she would have insisted they pay her more for rental allowance.

Guaranteed Pay

Guaranteed pay means that the hospital has an agreement with the agency to pay you for 36 to 40 hours regardless of whether the hospital uses you or not. The reason for this agreement is to ensure that the hospital cannot send you home early for the day without pay.

You do not want to travel across the country only to be canceled or sent away on low census days. This is one way that travel nursing is different than local agency nursing. Guaranteed pay is a standard benefit with most agencies. However, make sure it is written in your contract.

ABOVE AVERAGE BENEFITS

Not all agencies offer the following benefits. They are offered over and above the standard package. If you want one of these benefits, start by choosing an agency that already offers it. In other words, these are not benefits that you negotiate for later. Definitions of the following benefits were obtained from various agencies in the industry.

Tax Plans

Different companies may offer different optional tax plans, which can be very confusing. After talking with several recruiters, I've tried to sort these plans out for you.

Basically, most of these plans allow you to enjoy your tax deductions early. Instead of waiting until the end of the year to deduct what you can as a traveler, they give you a certain amount of the money tax free, and then you do not claim it as a deduction at the end of the year. This way, you get to use the money sooner. If you decide not to participate in the plans, then they will tax all your money and you will claim your deductions at the end of the year.

125 Cafeteria Plan

This cafeteria plan has nothing to do with food. Visualize this plan as a buffet of additional insurance options. The agency still provides free insurance, with additional options such as cancer insurance or prepaid legal assistance. You choose from the options, and pay for it by allowing them to deduct the funds from your paycheck before taxes so you are not taxed for the money.

For example, this plan is good for the traveler who has health insurance provided, but needs an additional amount taken out of the paycheck to include family members on the health insurance plan. The amount would be deducted from their paycheck before taxes were taken out.

Tax Advantage Program

The tax advantage program is a government program that allows a traveler who is 75 miles from their permanent residence to earn approximately $5 per hour tax free. The agency pays a fee to be able to provide this benefit. They will take out approximately $182 out of your paycheck each week before taxes and then put it back in.

Normally, you would deduct this money at the end of the year for your daily living expenses. This program basically allows you to deduct the money as you make it, so you do not have to wait until the end of the year.

Cash Advantage Program

The cash advantage program is designed for the travelers staying close to home while on contract. Normally this person would miss out on the travel reimbursement option. Instead of separating the travel reimbursement, housing allowance, and other benefits from your pay, the agency adds it to your hourly rate. This way, you still get your travel reimbursement money along with the other standard benefits while working a local assignment.

International Placement

Some agencies staff only in the United States. However, more companies are starting to expand internationally.

Medical Staff

Some agencies staff their office with all medical personnel. This way your recruiter can relate to your issues, concerns, and situations while you are on assignment. They are often more prepared to help you when you are having problems.

NEGOTIABLE BENEFITS

Extra perks are little things that are not always offered, but can be negotiated. Keep these items in mind so you know what you can negotiate for.

License Reimbursement

If you are a nurse, some agencies will cover the cost for you to obtain a license in the state you will be working in. Other agencies will reimburse you, but only after you have completed a few assignments with them. The cost and requirements for licensure vary greatly for each state and change on a regular basis.

Referral Bonus

Referral bonuses can be quite profitable ($200 to $1000). If you refer a traveler to an agency, the agency will pay you money for sending them a traveler.

The referral pay is given at the completion of that traveler's assignment. The traveler must make it a point to tell their recruiter that they were referred, and then follow it up at the end of their assignment. Some agencies may overlook this detail unless you remind them. Some travelers get together and refer each other so they can split the bonuses. Although this is not how it is meant to work, it sometimes happens.

Completion Bonuses

Completion bonuses are not always offered. The hospital usually offers the completion bonus to the agency, and the agency is supposed to pass this bonus on to you. Make sure to ask if a completion bonus is offered for the assignment. Completion bonuses are just what they sound like: a lump sum of money is paid to you upon the completion of the assignment.

Read the small print in your contract. Know the bonus criteria. One traveler reported finishing her assignment and expecting a completion bonus. Later, she found out that she was not eligible for the completion bonus because she was sent home early a few times on her assignment. The completion bonus was contingent upon her completion of the assignment and a minimum of 40 hours a week. Therefore, she did not meet the hourly requirement, and did not receive her bonus.

Extension Bonus

Whenever you decide to remain on an assignment for a longer period of time than originally contracted, it is called an *extension*.

Always try to negotiate for more money if you are asked to extend. Request either a bonus, or more money per hour. The hospital usually prefers to pay you more money rather than take the time to orient a new person. If the agency will not offer you more money, consider switching agencies for your extension if they will pay you more.

Education Reimbursement

Some agencies offer continuing education units through their company. Others may reimburse you for your own educational efforts.

LONG-TERM INCENTIVES

Long-term incentives are for those people who want to get maximum financial benefits from traveling by staying with one company.

While you gain financially, you may lose your choices of location. You must choose from the assignments the agency has available. If you want to stay with one agency, try to sign up with a larger company that will have plenty of assignments or a company that tends to specialize in the areas you like. Take the time to shop around before picking a long-term company. The investigative time will pay off.

Vacation Packages

You are not paid for the time off between assignments. Some agencies offer paid vacation packages after you work with them for a specific length of time, however.

401(k) Plans

Some 401(k) programs are effective immediately, and some are effective after you have been with the company a specified length of time. If you are thinking about staying with one company for all your travel assignments, be sure to inquire about their 401(k) activation time. These programs are good if you plan on working with one company full time for an extended period, and are one of the best retirement investment options available.

Overall, it is possible to have all the benefits of a permanent employee, and more. You may want to consult an accountant or financial planner regarding tax and retirement planning. Roth IRAs (individual retirement accounts) and other financial incentive programs are available to self-employed persons.

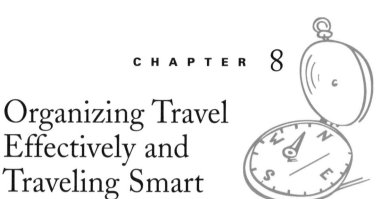

CHAPTER 8

Organizing Travel Effectively and Traveling Smart

Once you have accepted an assignment, your main challenge becomes that of staying organized in the midst of constant change. It is not easy living in several places during a single year. Sometimes you feel as if you are living out of your car. Amazingly, however, while you are on the road you are still able to find that missing document the agency needs.

Besides packing, the three main things in your life that need some thought and organization are mail, money, and human contact. There are several ways to organize each of these items. You have to choose the option that best fits your life.

MAIL

You have a few different options for what to do about your mail. This decision depends greatly on your current situation. The main objective is to manage your bills and pay them on time.

Forward Address at the Post Office

Many travelers forward their address to their new location each time they move. The disadvantage to this option is the paper trail you leave behind for the post office to figure out. This means you may get your mail late, and consequently your bills may arrive and be paid late.

If you have only a few bills, you can call the billing agencies directly and give them a change of address. One traveler, Penny, is lucky enough to have only one credit card bill. She does not worry much about her mail. She calls the credit card company at the beginning of each month and asks them for her new balance. Then she forwards the mail just in case she forgets something. Another traveler, Paul, says he pays extra on his bills just before he moves so the mail has time to catch up to him.

Forward Address to a Friend or Relative for Pick-up

If you have permanent home address, you can have a friend pick up your mail once a week. If the friend or family member cannot pick up your mail, you can have your mail forwarded to their house. This friend can call you with the information, or send your mail to you. Of course, the friend needs to be one who is dependable and trustworthy. For example, many travelers have all their mail forwarded to their parents. Then mom or dad either mails, calls, or e-mails them the information they need to know.

Get a Mailbox or Post Office Box

If you don't want to bother anyone with your mail, you can get a mailbox at places such as Mailboxes Etc., Mail Depot, or Mailco. These stores are privately owned, so their prices vary from store to store. Boxes usually range from $30 to $40 for 3 months or $80 to $90 dollars for 1 year. This is the price for a small box, which is all you need. The store will still hold your mail even if it does not fit in the box.

You simply call the mailbox place each time your address changes, and they forward your mail to your new address. Mailboxes Etc., for example, also allows you to call and ask them what is in your box. One advantage to using such a company is that your address is not a post office box number. The address appears more professional because it is usually a street address with a suite number attached. You may also rent a box at your local post office; for small boxes, the rate is around $26 for 6 months and $52 for 1 year.

MONEY

Before leaving, take some time to figure out how the money is going to get to your bank and how you are going to get the money out. You do not want to be in a strange state without money. If possible, carry a credit card and an ATM card for possible emergencies. You may want to make sure your money is in a bank with several locations throughout the country, especially if you plan on traveling for a while. Many travelers recommend Bank of America and Wells Fargo.

Direct Deposit

Often, health travel agencies have direct deposit. Direct deposit eliminates many hassles. A few agencies offer the benefit of providing local checks regardless of where you are located.

Mail in Deposits

If you do not live paycheck to paycheck, you can mail your deposit to the bank. They will give you a special address for this.

Banking Online

Finally, with the advancement of computers and computer banking, it is possible to pay all your bills via computer. You can also keep in touch with your friends via e-mail and save a lot of money in long distance calls.

PHONE

Set Up Phone Line Ahead of Time

Once you have the address of your new place from the housing agent, you may want to call and set up a phone line. This way, you already have a phone number and can give it to your friends before you leave.

Go Cellular

Now people also have the option of getting a one-rate plan on their cell phone. This allows you to keep a local phone number so it is not long distance for your friends back home to call. Plus, you do not pay for long distance charges when you call long distance. You pay one flat rate per month for a designated amount of minutes.

Some one-rate plans cost around $119 for 1000 minutes per month and $89 for 600 minutes per month. You pay the same rate whether your calls are long distance or not. This way, you can also keep a consistent phone number when you travel. Your phone goes where you go. Your long distance phone bill would probably cost as much as the cellular plan does anyway. Keeping track of your talk time is the main disadvantage to using a cell phone.

You may want to get a separate landline for Internet access, unless you want to pay the money for special laptop accessories. The accessory allows you to use your cell phone as an Internet access line. This option may cost as much as $500, however.

Calling Online

Did you know that you can make long distance calls online for virtually nothing? The reception is not the best, but it works. All you need is a set of headphones. The web site address is www.phonepad.com.

WHAT TO PACK

Most agencies provide basic furniture, and that's all. Bring anything else you "cannot live without." You will need all your necessities. The following is a list of the essentials:

1. Kitchen supplies
2. Reminders of home

3. Any hobby materials
4. Towels
5. Portable alarm clock
6. A folder with important papers and travel documents
7. A phone
8. Camera
9. Uniforms
10. Casual clothes
11. One formal or semi-formal outfit
12. Iron
13. Bed linens and a pillow
14. A shower curtain (optional)
15. Address book with all your friends
16. Map of where you are going
17. TV or microwave (optional, may not need it; ask)
18. Radio
19. Medications
20. Bank card
21. Extra check books
22. Pet (not impossible)
23. Laptop computer or palm device

You would be amazed how much fits into your car. Regardless of how much stuff you bring, you will need to take a trip to the nearest Wal-Mart, K-Mart, Target, or the like. You will invariably need basics, like toilet paper and laundry detergent.

Another alternative suggested by travelers is to arrive at your assignment location on a Friday, and go to the local garage sales on Saturday. You can find good deals on household items.

Bringing a pet is not impossible. Make sure to let the agency know ahead of time that this is a requirement you have. The agency will be responsible for finding housing that allows pets. A pet deposit is usually required.

TRAVELING SMART

Being organized is a good start, but what else do you need to know about traveling? After interviewing several travelers, the following suggestions were revealed:

1. Schmooze the housing agent. They are the ones that can get what you want in your apartment.
2. Negotiate, negotiate, negotiate.

3. Always get more money for an extension

4. Whenever possible, go somewhere you can stay with family or friends so you can pocket the housing money.

5. Anyone can set up a Federal Express account, Allen says. "It has saved me a lot of time and money. If I want something sent to me right away, like my paycheck, I give them my account number and let them bill it to me."

6. Find out what other companies will offer to pay you to work in the area you are planning on going. This way, you know if your agency is offering you an acceptable rate.

7. Make sure to get a contract signed before you leave, or you may get paid differently than what you were told on the phone.

8. Network with other travelers.

9. When you arrive at the apartment complex, be sure to do a walk through, making notes as you go. Give your written notes about anything wrong with the apartment to the manager.

10. Contact your company as soon as you know you want to extend your contract. This allows them time to reserve your housing so you do not have to switch apartments when you extend.

CONTRACT TIPS

If the hospital no longer wants you, they can terminate the contract at any time. If your contract is terminated, you will probably have only 24 hours to move out of the apartment. Make sure the termination clause is specified in the contract. Termination of a contract can happen. Some people fit into different environments better than others. If you are terminated from an assignment, it usually is due to personality conflicts rather than skill. You are a skilled, experienced professional and that is why they want you.

Read the Small Print

Sometimes, in the small print of your contract, the agency will specify whether or not you can become a permanent staff member at your assigned location. You may have to wait a year before applying for permanent placement at a facility in which you are a traveler.

Staying On

What if you want to extend your assignment at the same facility, but with a different company? Once again, read the small print. Your contract may state that you cannot work at that facility through another agency for a designated period of time.

At the end of your contracted time, you can switch to another company that the hospital is also using and negotiate with that new company for more benefits than you are currently receiving. This happens all the time. It can be done as long as you have not signed something saying you would not switch to another company.

Do not worry. Many companies don't have such policies. Several of them actually encourage permanent placement. However, you need to be aware of what to look for and what you may be getting into if you do not take the time to read the small print.

Ask Questions

Some policies are never mentioned to you verbally unless you ask. When a "what if" question comes to mind, ask it. Have them put it in writing.

For example, do they provide professional liability for you while you travel? Because you are a traveler, liability can become a gray area. Is the hospital responsible to cover you, or is the agency?

In another example, a company may state that they provide a 401(k) plan after you have worked for them full time for 6 months. Ask them to define exactly what they mean by "full time."

TRAVEL AND SAFETY

Use Your Brain

Independent-type people tend to cope best with being away from home. Many times, you may not have anyone else to rely on. You have to be resourceful and know how to be safe. One nurse, Adrian, shares her experience. She had just arrived to her new assignment. After completing a full day, she managed to find the grocery store in town. When she got ready to leave the store, she realized she had lost her keys. They were nowhere to be found. She was stuck in a new town on a Sunday afternoon with no keys and nobody to call. She called the local rental car agency, but they did not have a copy of the keys. A man offered her a ride, but she declined, knowing better than to put herself in a vulnerable situation. She took a cab to the apartments, where the apartment manager opened her door and provided an extra key. The next morning, she jogged to work and negotiated a deal with the rental car company.

Find Out Crime Information Before You Leave

Camie explains her safe approach to finding her travel destination. She finds out the name and address of her new apartment as soon as possible. Then she looks up the apartment complex online for more details. Next, she calls the police department to get the latest crime statistics in the area. Finally, she calls the Visitors Bureau in the area to ask if they know anything about the neighborhood. Also, she has them mail information to her new address about what to do in the area. When she arrives, she has a package of wonderful ideas and a map of the city.

Plan the Trip

Make sure to sit down and map out the way you plan on getting to your destination. Take into consideration such things as the weather, scenery, safety, and time. Tell someone your plan before you go.

Cathy, an experienced traveler, describes her first time on a road trip. "You are so out on your own," Cathy says. "You arrive in a town where you don't know anyone. When I tried to find my apartment for my first assignment in Baltimore, I got lost in a run-down neighborhood. I was terrified and shaking. Here I was in my brand new red convertible with Iowa license plates. Luckily, I had a map with me. I found the street nearest to me. Then, I just stayed on that street until I was finally out of that area."

Bring Emergency Supplies

Do not overlook the importance of bringing emergency supplies. You never know what situations may arise. A cell phone is recommended. The one-rate plan is wonderful for traveling. If you cannot afford service for the phone, that is okay too. Recently, a traveler shared this tip. She says the law requires wireless phone companies to keep 911 activated on cell phones even if the phone has no service. As long as you keep the phone charged, you can still reach the emergency number.

With as much traveling as you will be doing, it is a good idea to have a membership with the Automobile Association of America (AAA) or a Driver's 1 card (800-846-4000). Also, many automobile insurance companies now offer roadside assistance as a service. When driving, you have to take precautions. Do not allow yourself to get into a situation on the road that can be avoided. Have a plan for roadside assistance, and make sure to get your car checked, tire pressure equalized, and oil changed before leaving on a long trip. Also, carry an air pump for your tire that plugs into the cigarette lighter in case you get a flat tire in the middle of nowhere. The pump is inexpensive and can be found at stores like Wal-Mart, K-Mart, or Target.

Travel With a Friend

Try not to travel alone, especially if you are female. Traveling alone is not recommended, for obvious reasons. You never know what will happen. Find a friend who wants to go with you and enjoy the drive together. Find out how much it will cost if your friend needs to fly back. Purchasing a 21-day advance fare round-trip ticket is often significantly cheaper than a one-way ticket.

Take Your Time

Please take time to enjoy your trip to your assignment. Give yourself at least a week to drive. The drive is the beginning of your exciting journey, and there are things to see along the way. You are cheating yourself if you plow through the trip and never stop to smell the roses.

Travel Cheap

The agency usually offers you travel money. They pay you so many cents per mile up to a maximum total. Usually, the limit is gracious and should cover your expenses unless you are going a long distance, such as Alaska or Hawaii. As a matter of fact, if you are willing to camp out or stay at inexpensive hotels (such as Motel 6 or Red Roof Inn) on your travels, you can actually make money getting to your destination. Of course, be sure to check the area for safety, park in a well-lighted area, and trust your intuition. Some dedicated travelers travel in an RV. The agency pays you the same amount of travel allotment whether or not you spend it all or not.

Also, ask the hotels if they offer discounts to medical professionals. One traveler was on the road with her boyfriend, who owned a travel agency. As a travel agent, he was entitled to special discounts. While booking the room, her boyfriend jokingly asked if they gave discounts to nurses. Surprisingly, they said "yes" and gave them an even larger discount.

Travel Light

Try to bring as little as possible. You will get tired of moving it all every 3 months. One traveler says she ships most of her items, because it costs her only about $40 dollars to send 150 pounds through United Parcel Service.

ORIENTATION

Be Easygoing

Depending on your experience level, the first assignment can be difficult. Your orientation is short. Travelers must be flexible and have the ability to adapt to new situations quickly. It will make your life much easier to "go with the flow." Do things the employer's way, unless it is harmful to patient safety.

Particular institutions have their own personality and worldview on even the smallest things. They often think their way is the only way. You will be much happier if you take time to note the norms of the workplace and follow them, instead of trying to blaze new trails on trivialities. One nurse expressed it perfectly when she said, "You know your way, and then you learn their way."

Be a Survivalist

Usually, you are leaving everything that you currently know, to encounter all new experiences. When you arrive at the hospital, it is rare that someone will walk you through the process. You must take the initiative. When you don't know something, do not hesitate to ask someone.

Figure out exactly what resources you have in that setting. Who should you contact if something comes up? What phone numbers would be helpful to have handy? Where are things located? Try to take time to tour the unit by yourself on the first day. Look in every cabinet and place you can think of to get yourself acquainted with your environment.

Be Friendly

The sooner you make friends, the better off you will be. The staff can make your life miserable if they do not like you. Depending on where you go, the staff may be receptive to travelers or they may not. You will run across people who are jealous and resentful that you are a traveler.

Sometimes, travelers are assigned to the worst cases or patients in the department. For example, in surgery, the traveler sometimes is put in with the doctors that nobody likes to work with or is left to take care of the sickest patients. This sort of treatment is not the norm, but unfortunately, it does happen.

Until people get used to you and your skills, they may treat you like a novice. This can be frustrating for an experienced nurse. Remember to go with the flow, and things will be better after the first week.

Be Patient With Yourself

The first week is the worst. Major adjustments are going on. At first, you may feel like a new graduate or wonder how you forgot everything you learned.

Stress has amazing physical effects on the brain and on stamina. Suddenly, the simplest things are difficult because you do not know where everything is or who to call. It is analogous to doing your old job in the dark. Have you ever heard yourself say, "I could do this with my eyes closed?" Now is your chance. Eat well, take vitamins, and get plenty of rest.

WORKING A STRIKE

Strikes are a touchy subject. Both sides can argue a valid point. This section is not meant to encourage or discourage anyone about working strikes. The purpose of this section is to provide information so you can make informed decisions.

Earning Potential

You can make $35 to $50 an hour, depending on your specialty.

Agency Staffing

There are three agencies that mainly staff strikes: Travel Nurse International, HPO Staffing, and Faststaff.

States

The states most likely to have strikes seem to be California, Connecticut, Florida, Kentucky, Massachusetts, Michigan, Mississippi, New York, Ohio, Oregon, Pennsylvania, Nevada, New Jersey, Rhode Island, Vermont, and Washington, as well as Washington, D.C.

Strike Assignment Work Compared to Conventional Travel

The minimum commitment time during a strike assignment is usually 1 to 2 weeks. Often, you are guaranteed 48 hours of work per week. You have to be available immediately if you plan on working a strike. Strikes can be over just as soon as they start. If you fly to a strike and it settles while you are on your way, the company usually pays you $250 to $500 for making the attempt.

Twelve-hour shifts are not uncommon. This is especially profitable in California, where they pay time and a half for any time worked over 8 hours in one day.

You are usually put up in a hotel with a roommate who works an opposite shift from you. Almost all the other nurses you work with are also travelers. You meet nurses from all over the country and the bond is tight.

An element of danger does exist; however, safety measures are put in place to protect the nurse. Nurses are bused in together. The hospital usually has an emergency number to call if you feel you are being harassed.

The most important thing to watch out for is your patient. Sometimes, charts have been switched and IV pumps locked to make your life more difficult. Get to know your patients and double check orders, especially on the first day of work.

Working with agencies during a strike can be frustrating because the demand is so sudden. The agency scrambles to make so much happen at once. You may feel lost in the shuffle. Your recruiter is often difficult to contact. You may be left waiting for days without an answer about whether you will work. Meanwhile, you keep your local job on hold to make sure you are available at a moment's notice. The needs of the hospital during a strike change daily. Your file is sent to the hospital, and the hospital then decides whether or not to accept you based on their current needs.

The next thing you know, you may get a call from the agency at 10 at night to let you know you are scheduled to fly out of town early the next morning. It all happens too slowly in the beginning, and too fast in the end.

Expect the unexpected. You may arrive late and tired, and be sent to orientation before you ever see your hotel room. You may have sent all your papers to the agency, and arrive to find out that your file never made it to the site. You never know what can happen.

Strike Tips

1. When you turn in your time sheet, make sure to note your hourly rate at the bottom.
2. With your final time slip, write a reminder about your license reimbursement. Also, remind them not to tax the reimbursement money.
3. If you were there and available to work, but the hospital did not need you that day, write it down on the time slip. Sometimes you will be paid for being available. You cannot help that the hospital did not use you.
4. Always carry your nursing license with you.
5. Bring two complete copies of your file with all your current documents.
6. Be flexible and super meticulous about your documentation.
7. Take your vitamins. Nurses find that taking vitamins during a strike really helps them keep up their energy level and keep from getting sick while working so many hours.
8. Keep a financial goal in mind to help you get through the rough times.

No matter what type of assignment you are taking, planning ahead can make a difference in the experience you will have. Take note of these tips. These suggestions may seem simple, but they often have been learned the hard way.

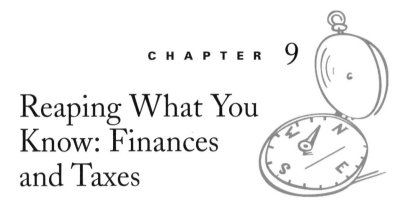

CHAPTER 9

Reaping What You Know: Finances and Taxes

While the earning potential of a traveler is great, the earning potential of a prepared traveler is greater. Strategically planning can make a big difference. This chapter is intended to increase your awareness of the tax benefits available to you when traveling and how to maximize those benefits. The financial strategy for traveling can be narrowed down to the three steps described in this chapter: maintain a permanent residence; find a good accountant; and stay informed.

ESTABLISH AND MAINTAIN A PERMANENT RESIDENCE

If at all possible, establish a permanent residence. Without a permanent residence, you will not be able to claim most of the tax deductions you can take advantage of as a traveler.

Most travel nursing agencies send you a form asking for your permanent address. A permanent residence does not have to be a place that you own. You can pay rent somewhere while you are gone even if the rent is $25 a month.

In 1999, the Internal Revenue Service (IRS) redefined "temporary work location" (Department of the Treasury, 1999). In general, employment at a work location is temporary if it is realistically expected to last for 1 year or less.

You are considered to be traveling away from home if your duties require you to be away from your tax home (permanent residence) longer than an ordinary day's work and to sleep overnight away from home to meet the demands of your work. (See IRS Publication 521, revised January 4, 2000.)

FIND A KNOWLEDGEABLE ACCOUNTANT

When traveling, your tax situation changes drastically. You have the opportunity to deduct much more than you would normally. Using an accountant is one major way you can maximize the financial benefits of traveling.

After a lengthy search, an accountant firm was located in San Diego that files hundreds of taxes for travelers per year. Karen Lutz and Dennis Hicks at Hicks Financial were kind enough to provide an interview. Dennis filed taxes for his first traveling nurse in 1995. "That traveling nurse actually taught me how to prepare such a return," says Dennis. "Now she continues to refer travelers to me. Each year I learn something new." Dennis owns the firm and Karen handles the taxes for many of the traveling nurse clients. The following are their responses to a few pertinent tax questions for travelers.

What Is Considered a Travel Assignment?

Any assignment that is more than 50 miles from your home and less than 12 months in duration is considered a travel assignment, as long as you stay overnight at the location of your assignment and maintain a permanent residence elsewhere.

In other words, if you are living at home and driving 50 miles to work every day and then driving back home, you are not officially, for tax purposes, working a travel assignment. Therefore, if you take an assignment in your hometown, you will not be eligible for all the tax deductions available to other travelers. The travel contract is the first step necessary to begin an assignment and should be included with your tax paperwork.

What Is Needed for Proof of Permanent Residency?

1. Car registration
2. Bank account
3. Voter registration
4. Property owner

Not all this information is necessary, but the more proof you can gather, the better. The number one item the IRS would most likely dispute is your permanent residency.

If you end up buying a new car while on assignment, it is recommended that you register the car in your home state next time you visit. Otherwise, the IRS may find it confusing as to where you live.

Even if you are renting an apartment from a relative or friend back home, make sure to send money home each month as evidence of maintaining a residency.

Does a Nurse Need to Return Home Sometime During the Year?

You don't have to return home to show proof of residency. It is recommended that you move on to a new travel assignment within 12 months.

Even if you stay in the same area, you should change assignments (hospital location). It is not necessary to change the employer (agency) as long as you change the location.

How Does State Tax Work When You Travel?

Basically, you are responsible for state taxes in your home state and in your travel state. The good news is that your home state tax will be offset by the tax you paid in the travel state. Therefore, you are credited and not taxed twice.

The only time you would not owe state tax is when neither your home nor your travel state has a state tax charge. The states that are free of state tax are Alaska, Florida, Nevada, New Hampshire, New Mexico, South Dakota, Tennessee, Texas, Washington, and Wyoming. Therefore, if you lived in Texas and took an assignment in Alaska, you would not owe any state tax.

The second most ideal situation would be to live and travel in states that charge less state tax. California, Hawaii, New York, Pennsylvania, Virginia, and Maryland, as well as the District of Columbia, tend to charge a higher state or local tax than most other states.

Keep in mind that state tax is only one consideration with regard to finances. Sometimes, the states with high state tax also pay more in wages.

What Sort of Things Can a Travel Nurse Deduct?

1. RN license fees (in any state)
2. Uniforms and shoes
3. Cell phones
4. Computer
5. Internet expenses
6. Continuing education
7. Malpractice insurance
8. Dues and subscriptions (e.g., AAA, nurse magazines)
9. Job search costs (e.g., airfare, faxes, Federal Express, medical tests)
10. Parking fees and tolls
11. Cost of shipping vehicles for assignments out of the country
12. Dry cleaning of uniforms
13. Long distance calls
14. Airfare expenses to visit home during an assignment
15. Cost of maintaining a post office box and postage

What About Reimbursements Such as Travel?

Most employers reimburse for travel expenses. Therefore, travel is deductible only if your employer does not reimburse you.

Keep in mind that the company should not be taxing you on any money that is a reimbursement, unless you have not adequately proven permanent residency in another location. The company should not tax you on the any reimbursements because they can deduct that money at the end of the year.

You can deduct any money you spend over and above the reimbursement, however. For example, if you pay $600 to fly to your assignment and the company reimburses you $400, you can deduct the $200 difference. The same goes for housing. If you find your own housing, and the company pays you $700 a month for a housing subsidy, but you pay $1000 rent a month, you can deduct $300 a month for housing ($3600 for the year) at the end of the year.

It really helps the accountant if you can total your expenses and total your reimbursements for the year. (For example: $1000 × 12 months for housing + utilities + airfare [or drove 1000 miles] + hotel costs, and note the number of days you were on the road.) Once you have a total of the expenses for the year, total the reimbursements you received from the company. Then subtract the total reimbursements from the total expenses.

Some companies will actually give you a 1099 form that reports all the reimbursements they gave you for the year that were not directly in your paycheck. Other companies designate what part of your pay was a reimbursement on the paycheck stub. Keep your paycheck stubs.

Can Nurses Deduct for Moving Expenses?

Some nurses want to deduct the cost of "moving" their belongings. Keep in mind that your travel is supposed to be temporary, so you should not have a moving van. Be careful what terminology you use. If you "moved," then how could you be a "traveler"? This sets up a whole different situation for tax purposes. The same goes with wanting to deduct storage expenses at home. You are supposed to be maintaining two households. Storage is not a household. However, you can deduct the expense of shipping a few boxes to your new assignment with items you couldn't fit in your car.

What If You Own a House in a Foreign Country?

You cannot deduct expenses associated with owning a home in another country on a U.S. tax return.

What If You Are Renting Out Your House Back Home?

Owning a home in the United States is great because you can deduct the expenses associated with the house as well as all the travel deductions.

However, you cannot deduct the house as a rental. Why? Because if you are renting out your home, then how can you be maintaining it as your residence and claiming to be a traveling nurse? If you rent out a home, you are not maintaining a home.

What About Working as an Independent Contractor?

Working as an independent contractor on an assignment is very questionable. Proving yourself as an independent contractor to the IRS can be tricky. If you do decide to work as an independent contractor, you better make sure you are getting paid considerably more. Since you become both the employee and the employer, you owe social security tax for both. This can turn out to be around 15% of your earnings.

What Documents Make Life Easier for the Accountant?

1. Receipts for anything deductible
2. Copy of your travel contracts for the year
3. A log of where you have been and the dates

Besides the Obvious, How Can an Accountant Be Helpful?

In the event the IRS audits you, never go by yourself if you can avoid it. Let an experienced professional properly prepare your documentation. In the long run, the expense will far outweigh the final outcome of an audit. Most audits are done by mail now anyway. Keep your records for at least 5 years.

STAY WELL INFORMED

Accountants can educate you. The more educated you are about your own tax situation, the less taxes you will pay.

With today's e-mail and faxes, you can send your tax information to anyone throughout the world to prepare your taxes. Be sure to make copies of all the information before you send it. If you cannot get your information together by the April 15 deadline, just have your accountant file an extension. In most situations, if you are receiving a refund, you have up to 3 years to file without a penalty. The penalty after 3 years is a forfeit of your refund.

While having an accountant is important, it is also important to stay well informed yourself. Did you know that your food and living expenses are tax deductible while working away from home? You can collect all your receipts on an assignment and give them to your accountant at the end of the year.

If collecting receipts sounds like a big headache, you can deduct a daily standard meal allowance. For travel in 2000, the meal allowance rate was $30 to $46 a day and the lodging allowance was approximately $55 per day, depending on where and when you travel. (See IRS Publication 1542, April 2000, for the specific allowance of each city and state.) You can deduct the standard meal allowance whether you are an employee or self-employed. Your accountant will have this information. However, if you want to find out for yourself, you can find the information on the Internet at www.policyworks.gov/perdiem.

Standard meal allowances for areas outside the continental United States are published monthly in the *Maximum Travel Per Diem Allowances for Foreign Areas*. Your employer may have these rates available or you can purchase the publication from the Superintendent of Documents, U.S. Government Printing Office, P.O. Box 371954, Pittsburgh, PA 15250-7954, or order it by calling 1-202-512-1800.

Also, note how much your company is paying you per mile for travel. If they are not paying you the standard mileage deduction, you can claim the difference at the end of the year. For 2000, the standard mileage deduction was 32.5 cents per mile. This rate is adjusted periodically. (See IRS Publication 505, January 4, 2000.) If you traveled and the agency paid you only 25 cents per mile, you can deduct 7.5 cents (32.5 − 25 = 7.5) per mile at the end of the year.

Claiming a permanent residence and staying up on the latest tax laws is the key. The tax laws are constantly changing. Many tips are passed along by word of mouth, and aren't always accurate. *Caution:* You must verify all tax advice with your accountant or the IRS.

Some agencies recommend calling the National Enrolled Agents for tax advice at 1-800-424-4339 (fax 301-990-1611). You can also contact the Internal Revenue Service directly at 1-800-829-1040 or research their web site at www.irs.gov. Scroll down to the bottom of the web site and click on "Pubs and Forms." Publication numbers 593 and 54 have tax information about traveling abroad. If you are considering independent contracting, you may want to look at Publication number 533.

Other IRS publications pertinent to travelers include the following:

Business expenses: publications 17, 334, 529, 535
Travel expenses: publication 463
Moving expenses: publication 521
Education expenses: publication 508
Medical expenses: publication 502
Per diem rates: publication 1542 (revised April 2000)

Recently, a traveler named Kevin mentioned an unusual tax tip. Kevin says travelers are starting to share the idea of establishing an incorporated business. The traveler has the agency pay their business. Then the traveler pays himself a salary out of the business. This way, he or she is eligible for additional business deductions. Meanwhile, the traveler can divide the money between himself and the business in order to stay in a lower tax bracket. This idea needs to be explored further. Travelers recommend reading *Incorporate and Grow Rich! How to Cut Your Taxes 70% and Protect Your Assets Forever!* by C.W. Allen, C. Hill, and G. Sutten.

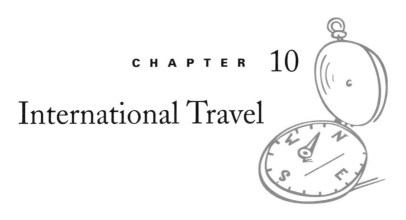

CHAPTER 10

International Travel

International travel is "the future of nursing," says Gary Fanger, founder and owner of Travel Nurse International. The nursing shortage is not expected to improve anytime soon. Bringing nurses to the United States from other countries is not the answer to the shortage, but it can help while other solutions are put into place.

In general, foreign nurses want to work in the United States for its money-making potential. Nurses in the United States are so stressed from the shortage that many of them want to travel outside the country for the adventure and excitement, even if it means less money. Let's face it: the grass is always greener on the other side, isn't it?

IMMIGRATING TO THE UNITED STATES

Currently, becoming a nurse in the United States is a long and tedious process. According to Carl Shusterman, an immigration attorney specializing in foreign nurses and physicians, the current immigration process can take as long as 18 months.

Finding a Sponsor

If you want to work in the United States, you must first find a sponsor. Refer to Appendix C to find staffing agencies involved in foreign travel.

Taking English Proficiency Exams

If you graduated from an English-speaking school, you may be exempt from the English exams. Most exempt nurses are from Australia, Canada (except Quebec), Ireland, New Zealand, and the United Kingdom. All other nurses must complete one of the following sets of English language proficiency exams:

Exams Administered by the Educational Testing Service
(ETS, 1-609-771-7100)
1. Test of English as a foreign language (TOEFL), $110,
   www.toefl.org
2. Test of written English (TWE)
3. Test of spoken English (TSE)

Exams Administered by the English Language Institute
(ELI, 1-734-763-3452)
1. Parts 1 to 3 of the Michigan English Language Assessment
2. Oral interview section

Taking the NCLEX

When you have completed the certification of the Commission on
Graduates of Foreign Nursing Schools (CGFNS), most states allow
you to apply for a temporary nursing license. Once you are in the
United States, you can take the National Council Licensure Examina-
tion (NCLEX), which is offered in most U.S. locations on a daily basis.
The NCLEX is the United States nursing exam. Once the NCLEX is
passed, it never expires and can be used to apply for any state licensure.
Information about licensure requirements for different states can be
found at the web site for the National Council of State Boards of
Nursing (www.ncsbn.org).

Usually, when you apply for a license in the desired state, the nursing
board sends you the information you need to take the NCLEX. You cannot take the exam without first applying for a license in a particular state.
When you go to take the NCLEX, you will be asked which state you
have applied for licensure. It doesn't matter which state you apply with,
as long as you apply with one.

NCLEX (National Council of State Boards of Nursing)
676 N. St. Clair
Suite 550
Chicago, IL 60611
800-551-1912
www.ncsbn.org

Information on studying for the exam can be found at www.nclex_rn.net
or www.nclex.com. The test is $120 dollars and is offered throughout the
United States (including the District of Columbia), American Samoa,
Northern Mariana Islands, Puerto Rico, and the Virgin Islands. Specific
test site locations can be found at www.2test.com.

Taking the CGFNS

If the NCLEX is not offered in a location near you, you may elect to take the CGFNS certification program. This program reviews your credentials and allows you to assess your chances of passing the U.S. registered nursing licensing exam (NCLEX-RN) by giving you an exam similar to the NCLEX. For immigration purposes, they will accept the NCLEX or CGFNS. However, in order to work, you will still have to take the NCLEX when you get to the United States.

Commission on Graduates of Foreign Nursing Schools
3600 Market Street
Suite 400
Philadelphia, PA 19104-2651
215-349-8767
support@cgfns.org or www.cgfns.org

The application fee for the CGFNS is $295 (includes study guide), reapplication is $250.

The CGFNS certification program is offered in the following countries: Australia (Perth and Sydney), Barbados (Bridgetown), Brazil (Rio de Janeiro), Canada (Montreal, Toronto and Vancouver), Egypt (Cairo), France (Paris), Germany (Frankfurt), Ghana (Accra), Hong Kong, Indonesia (Jakarta), Ireland (Dublin), Israel (Tel Aviv), Jamaica (Kingston), Japan (Tokyo), Jordan (Amman), Kenya (Nairobi), Korea (Seoul), New Zealand (Wellington), Pakistan (Karachi), Peru (Lima), Philippines (Manilla, Cebu City, Cagayan de Oro City), South Africa (Johannesburg), Sri Lanka (Colombo), Sweden (Goteborg), Switzerland (Geneva), Taiwan (Taipei), Thailand (Bangkok), United Kingdom (London), Guam (Agana). The CGFNS certification program also is offered in the United States: California (Los Angeles), Florida (Miami), Georgia (Atlanta), Hawaii (Honolulu), Illinois (Chicago), New York (New York), and Texas (Houston).

Applying for a Social Security Card

Once you arrive in the United States, you will receive an I-94 form at Immigration. Take the form, and apply for a social security number immediately at the local Social Security Administration office. You cannot get a paycheck until you have a social security number.

Social Security Administration
P.O. Box 17049
Baltimore, MD 21235
1-800-772-1213
www.ssa.gov

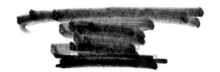

Obtaining an International Driver's License

Before you leave the United States, consider getting an international drivers license at the American Automobile Association (AAA; 800-922-8228 or 415-565-2012).

If you are arriving in the United States, most U.S. rental car companies require you to have an international driver's license and a credit card from an American bank. Check with your local passport center to find out how to get an international driver's license.

National Passport Center
P.O. Box 371971
Pittsburgh, PA 15250-7971
888-362-8668
http://travel.state.gov

Contacting the Local U.S. Consulate

Traveling nursing agencies should assist you with the immigration process. If you have further questions, however, you can contact your local U.S. consulate (www.arminco.com/embusa/consul.htm). More information on immigration can be found at 1-800-357-5283, www.ins.usdoj.gov, or www.us-immigration.com. Immigration forms can be downloaded from www.1mmigration.com.

Entering the United States at the Port of Entry

At the port of entry, U.S. government officials will inspect you. They will do four different inspections: public health, immigration, customs, and agriculture. You will be asked to provide your basic identification information, the address you will be staying in the United States, passport, and nursing credentials (certifications, nursing license in your country, CGFNS or NCLEX).

GOING TO THE UNITED STATES FROM CANADA

The North American Free Trade Agreement (NAFTA) makes it relatively easy for Canadians to work in the United States and for U.S. citizens to work in Canada.

Canadian nurses can work in the United States for 1 year. Annually, Canadians return to the border and cross again to renew their time in the United States. If you are Canadian, all you need to cross the border are the following:

Letter from your company, on their letterhead, stating your position, job description, hospital location, salary, and start date

- Birth certificate, ID, or passport
- Canadian RN license and U.S. RN license, if available
- At least $56 U.S. for crossing fees

Also, carry copies of all your medical documents and certifications for your nursing assignment.

If you have not taken the NCLEX yet, you can still work in one of the following states:

Alabama
Connecticut
Maine
Missouri
New Mexico
New York (1 year temporary permit)
North Carolina
Wisconsin

A few other states will accept the Canadian RN exam (CNAT) if you scored above 400 before a certain date. The date of the exam requirement varies from state to state. The states that seem to accept the CNAT exam, but with limitations as to when it was taken and the score, are: Alaska, California, Connecticut, Florida, Louisiana, Maryland, Massachusetts, New Hampshire, New Mexico, North Dakota, and Tennessee. All the states require Canadians to have attended an English-speaking school. If not, you must take the English proficiency exams. The CGFNS test locations in Canada are Montreal, Toronto, and Vancouver. The NCLEX can be taken across most state borders or in Manitoba, Canada.

TRAVELING OUTSIDE THE UNITED STATES

Working outside the United States is not usually a moneymaking venture, except in the Middle East. In general, nurses tend to make less money in other parts of the world. For example, the pay in the United Kingdom and Australia is approximately $27,000 to $36,000 (U.S.) per year. If you want to travel to another country, you may want to consider saving money and paying off bills before you go.

Plan on spending 6 to 8 months in processing before being able to travel. The process of proving your credentials and obtaining a visa still takes time, even though the U.S. nursing education is highly regarded in other countries.

It can be difficult to find companies that send nurses to other countries because there is not much money to be made in doing so. Even more difficult is finding a company that sends nurses to a country that speaks a foreign language.

If you are really serious about working outside the United States, apply for licensure in the country where you want to go. The licensure application is often the most difficult and tedious part of the process, and staffing companies will take you more seriously if you have applied.

Nursing Boards Outside the United States

Australia Nursing Council, Inc.
20 Chalis Street, First Floor
DICKSON ACT2602
+61 2 6257 7960
Fax: +61 2 6257 7955
www.anci.org.au
General information: anci@ancilorg.au
Overseas Information: overseas@anci.org.au

An Bord Altranais 31/32 (Irish Nursing Board)
Fitzwilliam Square
Dublin 2, Ireland
353-1-639-8500
Fax: 353-1-676-3348
www.nursingboard.ie/

United Kingdom Central Council for Nursing
23 Portland Place
London W1B1PZ
020 7637 7181
Fax: 020 7436 2924
www.ukcc.org.uk
More information on U.K. nursing immigration:
   www.nursingintheuk.co.uk

Virgin Islands Board of Nurse Licensure
P.O. Box 4247
St. Thomas, V.I. 00803
340-776-7397
Fax: 340-776-7131

College of Nurses of Ontario
101 Davenport Rd.
Toronto, Ontario
M5R3P1 Canada
416-928-0900
Fax: 416-928-6507
www.cno.org

Collegio Infermieri La Spezia (Italy)
Via Crispi 33
La Spezia
Italy 19125 Europe
+3918722247
Fax: +391877750584
www.ipasvi.laspezia.net

Additional Nursing Boards
American Samoa (684) 633 1222 206
Guam 011 (671) 475 0251
N. Mariana Islands 01 670 234 8950
Puerto Rico (787) 725 8161

Traveling to the Middle East

If you want a totally unique experience, you may want to consider traveling to Saudi Arabia. Mary traveled there and reports the inside scoop.

If you go to Saudi Arabia, the commitment is usually for 2 years. Vacation is once a year for approximately 30 days. You can always break the contract if you do not like it; you will just lose your bonus. The money is good because it is not taxed. Most companies pay around $36,000 to $38,000 a year, which is like making around $50,000 a year in the United States.

You live in an American compound and work at an American hospital. According to Mary, one of the best hospitals to work at is King Faisal Specialist Hospital and Research Center.

Inform yourself about cultural differences. Women must have their bodies covered so as not to show any curves or they can be taken to jail. A women must not be seen with any man in public unless he is related to her. Mary could have been in real trouble with her Arab boyfriend. She shares how she would sneak past the guards at her boyfriend's compound every week. Businesses shut down for 15 minutes during the day for prayer. During this time, she would sneak in to see her boyfriend. Although this makes for a great story, it is not recommended. Remember, you are subject to the laws of the area and their consequences. Review the laws of the culture and be sensitive to them. The consequences can be severe and are not worth the risk.

Another Middle Eastern area to travel to is United Arab Emirates. Their commitment requirement is for only 1 year, and the people there are more "westernized" than in Saudi Arabia.

If you are thinking about going to Saudi Arabia, read two books before you go, *Nine Hearts of Desire* and *Princess*. Also, watch the movie *Not Without My Daughter*.

SPECIAL TIPS FOR TRAVELING ABROAD

Make sure you have a signed, valid passport (and visa, if required). Fill in the emergency information page of your passport.

- If you get into trouble, contact the nearest U.S. embassy.
- Before you leave, note the contact information of the local embassy and emergency contact numbers (local police, hotel, fire department).
- Log onto http://travel.state.gov to find out any possible dangers, laws, and recommended immunizations for the place you plan to visit.
- Make two copies of your passport and any credit cards. Leave one copy with family, and carry the other copy separate from the originals.
- Do not leave your luggage unattended or wear flashy clothing or jewelry.
- Bring an extra pair of glasses and any medications you need. Bring a doctor's note for any narcotics you need to bring with you.
- Make sure your health insurance covers you abroad. Consider purchasing a short-term health and emergency assistance policy designed for travelers that includes evacuation in the event of an accident.

Bibliography

A new kind of nursing license for a new age of interstate practice. (2001). *HT, 8*(4), 49.

Bureau of Labor Statistics. (2000). *Occupational outlook*. Net Code 3502. Available at: http://www.bls.gov.

Dull, M. (1999). Developments in temporary staffing: Redefining the role of travel nurse agencies. *Nursing Watch, 3,* 7.

Ericksen, A. (2001). Shining in the OR. *HT, 8*(5), 9.

Johnson, T. *Job opportunities.* Princeton, NJ: Peterson's, 1999.

Schaffzin, N., & Bernstein, A. (1998). *Guide to your career.* New York: Random House.

Smith, D. (1995). Job satisfaction, productivity, and organizational commitment. JONA, 25(9), 17-25.

Thrailkill, D. (1999). *Executive temp.* New York: Random House.

U.S. Department of the Treasury. (1999). *Travel, entertainment, gift, and car expenses for 1999 returns* (463. Cat. No. 11081L). U.S. Government Printing Office 456-575.

Volunteer service organizations. (2001). *HT, 8*(4), 53.

Willard, J. (2000). Travel and registry nurses help fill staffing gaps. *Nursing Management, 31*(1), 46–47.

APPENDIX A

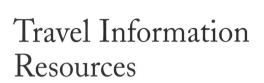

Travel Information Resources

MAGAZINES

Healthcare Traveler Magazine (HT)

A free magazine just for travelers. To order or change address, call 410-749-3200 or 1-800-9HT-TRAV, or visit the web site at: www.healthcaretraveler.com.

Travel Nursing 2000

A special edition for travelers put out by *Critical Nurse* every year in June.

Professional Journals

Staffing agencies advertise in the back of professional journals.

ONLINE INFORMATION

City Maps

www.mapblast.com
www.mapquest.com
www.citysearch.com

Discussion Groups for Travelers

Travelnursingcentral.com is a gathering point for travelers to share information, rank the quality of agencies, and obtain assistance in finding an assignment to fit their needs. It gives the traveler a chance to have a unified voice and support services. They can also be reached at 1-800-253-0774.

www.crosscountry.com has chat rooms and articles for travelers.
www.allnurse.com has discussion forums.
www.delphi.com (search: travel nursing) offers great travel tips.
www.scab.org has message boards and tips for nurses who work strikes.
A communication site for health care workers is available through:

Health Staff Australia Pty Ltd
A.B.N. 85 074 537 152
P.O. Box 373 Heidelberg Victoria 3084
AUSTRALIA
Phone: +61 3 9459 9999
Fax: +61 3 9458 4788
www.healthstaff.com.au

Airlines

The following web sites provide information about either specific airlines or fare information.

www.princeton.edu/Main/air800.html (airline phone numbers)
www.economytravel.com
www.lowestfare.com
www.expedia.msn.com
www.priceline.com
www.flifo.com
www.travelocity.com
www.cheaptickets.com
www.flyaow.com
www.4airline.com
www.aircanada.ca
www.aa.com
www.cdnair.ca
www.continental.com
www.delta-air.com
www.nwa.com
www.southwest.com
www.twa.com
www.ual.com
www.usairways.com

Taxes

Information on tax preparation and tax considerations for travelers can be found at the following companies or government agencies.

Hicks Financial Services
2240 Garnet Ave. Suite B
San Diego, CA 92109
Phone: 1-858-581-3336
Fax: 1-858-581-3375
www.hicksfinancial.com

National Enrolled Agents
200 Orchard Ridge Dr. #302
Gaithersburg, Maryland 20878
Phone: 800-424-4339
Fax: 301-990-1611

Internal Revenue Service

www.irs.gov
Publication 463: Travel
Publication 54: Taxes When Traveling Abroad
Publication 593: Highlights for Going Abroad
Publication 533: Self Employed

Health Insurance

Consider getting individual insurance, and get companies to reimburse you for your insurance rather than going on COBRA on the end of each assignment.

www.quotesmith.com
www.Healthaxis.com
www.unicare.com
www.usaa.com

Accommodations

Locate your own housing or look up the housing you're assigned before traveling.

www.apartments.com
www.rentnet.com
www.petplace.com (for pet-friendly hotels)

Nursing Boards Information

www.ncsbn.org lets you find the web site links to any nursing board in the United States and review updates on which states are now involved in the compact.

Education

For distance classes (RN and MSN programs), check the following.

University of Iowa
Center for Credit Programs
116 International Center
Iowa City, IA 52242-1802
Phone: 1-800-272-6430
www.uiowa.edu/~ccp

University at the Sea: earn CEUs while on a cruise
www.universityatsea.com

**The Sycamore Tree Center for Home Education
(home schooling children)**
2179 Meyer Place
Costa Mesa, CA 92627
Phone: 949-650-4466 or 1-800-779-6750
E-mail: 75767.1417@compuserve.com
www.sycamoretree.com

Location Information

General information: www.nettravelexchange.com (worldwide accommodations, maps, weather, and more)

Currency conversions for different forms of money: www.xe.com/ucc/

Chambers of commerce: www.chamberofcommerce.com (access to any chamber of commerce in the United States, to find out what to do in the area)

Cost of living: www.datamasters.com (analysis of cost of living in 400 U.S. cities)

Time zones: www.worldtimeserver.com (tells you, in real time, what time it is anywhere in the world)

Automobile Rentals

Alamo Rent-A-Car 800-327-9633
American International Rental Car 800-831-4118
Avis Rent-A-Car 800-831-2847
Bargain Car & Truck Rentals 800-874-1074
Budget Car & Truck Rental 800-527-0700
Courtesy Auto Rental 800-222-6741
Dependable Car Rental 800-522-3076
Dollar Rent-A-Car 800-800-4000
Enterprise Rent-A-Car 800-325-8007
Hertz Rent-A-Car 800-654-3131
National Car Rental Reservations 800-328-4567
Payless Car Rental 800-729-5377
Practical Atlas Car and Jeep Rental 800-367-5238
Rent-A-Wreck 800-535-1391
Sears Rent-A-Car 800-527-0770
Thrifty Car Rental 800-367-2277
Town & Country Car Rental 800-248-4350
U-Save Auto Rental of America Inc. 800-438-2300
Western Car Rental 800-231-5537
Information provided by Budget Rental Car 2000.

Hotel and Motel Toll Free Number

Best Western 800-528-1234
Budgetel 800-428-3438
Choice (Comfort Inn, Quality, Econolodge, Sleep) 800-446-6900
Clarion Hotel 800-221-2222
Comfort Inns 800-228-5150
Days Inn 800-325-2525
Downtowner Inns 800-251-1962
Econolodge 800-553-2666
Economy Inns of America 800-826-0778
Embassy Suites 800-362-2779
Four Seasons Hotels 800-268-6282
Friendship Inns 800-453-4511
Hilton International 800-445-8667
Holiday Inn 800-465-4329
Howard Johnson 800-654-2000
Hyatt Hotels & Resorts 800-233-1234
Knights Inn 800-843-5644
La Quinta 800-531-5900
Marriott Hotels Worldwide Reservations 800-228-9290
Master Host Inns 800-251-1962
Motel-6 800-466-8356
Omni Hotels Worldwide Reservations 800-843-6664
Quality Inns 800-228-5151
Radisson Hospitality Worldwide 800-333-3333
Ramada 800-272-6232
Red Carpet Inn 800-251-1962
Red Lion Inns 800-547-8010
Red Roof Inn 800-843-7663
Renaissance Hotels 800-468-3571
Rodeway Inns 800-228-2000
Sheraton Hotels 800-325-3535
Stouffer Hotels & Resorts 800-468-3571
Super-8 800-800-8000
Travelodge 800-578-7878
Westin Hotels 800-228-3000
Wyndam Hotels & Resorts 800-992-4326
Information provided by Budget Rental Car 2000.

State Board Nursing Information: Temporary

State	Fee	Expiration Time	Process Time*
Alabama 770 Washington Ave Suite 250 Montgomery AL 36104 334-242-4060 www.abn.state.al.us	$50	3 mon	5-10 days
Alaska 3601 C St. Suite 722 Anchorage, AK 99503 907-465-2544 www.dced.state.ak.us/occ/pnur.htm	$50	4 mon	WT
Arizona 1651 E. Morten Suite 150 Phoenix AZ 85020 602-331-8111 www.azboardofnursing.org	$25	4 mon	3-5 days
Arkansas 1123 S. University Ave Suite 800 Little Rock, AR 72204 501-686-2700 www.state.ar.us/nurse	$10	3 mon	1-2 days

State	Fee	Expiration Time	Process Time*
California 400 R Street Suite 4030 Sacramento CA 95815 916-322-3350 www.rn.ca.gov	$30	6 mon	4-6 wk by mail
Colorado 1560 Broadway Suite 670 Denver CO 80202 303-894-2430 www.dora.state.co.us/nursing	$85	4 mon	WT
Connecticut 410 Capital Ave. MS 12 HSR Hartford CT 06134 860-509-7624 www.state.ct.us/dph	$90	4 mon	7-10 days
Delaware 861 Silver Lake Blvd. Suite 203 Dover DE 19904 302-739-4522	$65	3 mon	WT
D.C. Boards 825 North Capitol Street Room 2224 Washington DC 20002 202-442-9200	$50	NA	4 wk
Florida 4080 Woodcock Drive 202 Jacksonville FL 32207 904-858-6940 www.doh.state.fl.us/mqa/nursing/rnhome.htm	$75	2 mon	10-15 days

State	Fee	Expiration Time	Process Time*
Georgia 166 Pryor Street, SW Atlanta GA 30303 404-656-3943 www.sos.state.ga.us/ebd-rn	$60	6 mon	15 days
Hawaii 1010 Richards St Honolulu HI 96801 808-586-3000	0	3 mon	WT
Idaho 280 N. 8th Street Suite 210 Boise ID 83720 208-334-3110 www.state.id.us/ibn/ibn/ibnhome.htm	$15	3 mon	WT
Illinois 100 West Randolph 9-300 Chicago, IL 60601 312-814-2715 www.dpr.state.il.us.	$25	6 mon	2 wk
Indiana 402 W. Washington St Room 041 Indianapolis IN 46204 317-232-2960 www.state.in.us/hpb	$10	3 mon	WT/48 hr
Iowa 1223 E. Court Ave Des Moines IA 50319 515-281-3255 www.state.ia.us/government/nursing	$78	1 mon	3-5 days

State	Fee	Expiration Time	Process Time*
Kansas 900 S W Jackson Street Suite 551-S Topeka KS 66612 785-296-4929 www.ink.org/public/ksbn	$70	4 mon	10 days
Kentucky 312 Whittington Pkwy 300 Louisville KY 40222 502-329-7000 www.kbn.state.ky.us	$70	6 mon	7-10 days
Louisiana 3510 N. Causeway Blvd 501 Metairie LA 70002 504-838-5332 www.lsbn.state.la.us	$50	3 mon	10 days
Maine 158 State House Station Augusta ME 04333 207-287-1133 www.state.me.us/pfr/auxboards/nurhome.htm	$60	3 mon	WT
Maryland 4140 Patterson Ave Baltimore MD 21215 410-585-1900 dhmh1d.dhmh.state.md.us/mbn	$25	3 mon	WT
Massachusetts 100 Cambridge Street Room 1519 Boston MA 02202 617-727-9961 www.state.ma.us/reg/boards/rn	$75	NA	6 wk

State	Fee	Expiration Time	Process Time*
Michigan 611 West Ottawa Lansing MI 48909 517-373-9102 www.cis.state.mi.us/bhser/genover.htm	$40	NA	Varies
Minnesota 2829 University Ave, SE 500 Minneapolis MN 55414 612-617-2270 www.nursingboard.state.mn.us	$50	6 mon	1 wk
Mississippi 1935 Lakeland Dr. Suite B Jackson MS 39216 601-987-4188	$25	3 mon	2 days
Missouri 3605 Missouri Blvd. Jefferson City MO 65102 573-751-0681 www.ecodev.state.mo.us/pr/nursing	$19	6 mon	WT
Montana 111 North Jackson Arcade Bldg., 4C Helena MT 59620 406-444-2071 www.com.state.mt.us/License/POL/index.htm	$70	3 mon	3-5 days
Nebraska P.O. Box 94986 Lincoln NE 68509 402-471-4376 www.hhs.state.ne.us/crl/nns.htm	$76	2 mon	WT

State	Fee	Expiration Time	Process Time*
Nevada 1755 East Plumb Lane 260 Reno NV 89502 775-688-2620 www.nursingboard.state.nv.us	$50	4 mon	2 wk
New Hampshire 78 Regional Dr Bldg. B Concord NH 03302 603-271-2323 www.state.nh.us/nursing	$20	6 mon	1 wk
New Jersey P.O. Box 45010 Newark NJ 07101 973-504-6586 www.state.nj.us/lps/ca/medical.htm	$50	NA	4-6 wk
New Mexico 4206 Louisiana NE Suite A Albuquerque NM 87109 505-841-8340 www.state.nm.us/clients/nursing	$90	6 mon	2 wk
New York Cultural Education Center Room 3023 Albany NY 12230 518-474-3843 www.op.nysed.gov/nurse.htm	$120	NA	8 wk
North Carolina 3724 National Dr. Raleigh NC 27602 919-782-3211 www.ncbon.com	$75	6 mon	WT; appointment

State	Fee	Expiration Time	Process Time*
North Dakota 919 South 7th St. Suite 504 Bismarck ND 58504 701-328-9777 www.ndbon.org	$75	3 mon	2 days
Ohio 77 South High St. 17th Floor Columbus OH 43266 614-466-3947 www.state.oh.us/nur	$50	4 mon	2 wk
Oklahoma 2915 N. Classen Blvd. Suite 524 Oklahoma City OK 73106 405-962-1800	$55	3 mon	Varies
Oregon 800 NE Oregon 465 Portland OR 97232 503-731-4745 www.osbn.state.or.us	$50	NA	1 wk
Pennsylvania 129 Pine St. Harrisburg PA 17101 717-783-7142 www.dos.state.pa.us/bpoa/nurbd/mainpage.htm	$20	1 yr	Varies
Rhode Island 3 Capitol Hill Cannon Bldg. Room 104 Providence RI 02908 401-222-3855	$75	3 mon	2 wk

State	Fee	Expiration Time	Process Time*
South Carolina 110 Centerview Dr. Suite 202 Columbia SC 29211 803-896-4550 www.llr.state.sc.us/bon.htm	$10	3 mon	WT
South Dakota 4300 S. Louise Ave. Suite C-1 Sioux Falls SD 57106 605-362-2760 www.state.sd.us/dcr/nursing	$15	3 mon	WT
Tennessee 425 5th Ave. North Cordel Hull Bldg. Nashville, TN 37247 615-532-5166 170.142.76.180/bmf-bin/BMFproflist.pl	$50	6 mon	4 wk
Texas 333 Guadalupe Suite 3-460 Austin TX 78701 512-305-7400 www.bne.state.tx.us	$15	12 wk	2 wk
Utah 160 E. 300 South Salt Lake City UT 84114 801-530-6628 www.commerce.state.ut.us	$50	NA	3 wk
Vermont 109 State St. Montpelier VT 05609 802-828-2396 vtprofessionals.org/nurses	$60	3 mon	WT

State	Fee	Expiration Time	Process Time*
Virginia 6606 West Broad St. 4th Floor Richmond VA 23230 804-662-9909 www.dhp.state.va.us	$50	1 mon	WT
Washington 1300 Quince St. SE Olympia WA 98504 360-236-4713 www.doh.wa.gov/hsqa/hpqad/Nursing	$40	NA	4 wk
West Virginia 101 Dee Drive Charleston WV 25311 304-558-3572 www.state.wv.us/nurses/rn	$10	3 mon	2 days
Wisconsin 1400 E. Washington Ave. Madison WI 53708 608-266-2112 www.state.wi.us	$10	3 mon	WT
Wyoming 2020 Carey Ave. Suite 110 Cheyenne WY 82002 307-777-7601 nursing.state.wy.us	$45	3 mon	10 days

WT, walk-through state; NA, not available.

*Money order or cashier's check usually speeds up the process.

†Source: All information changes regularly and must be verified. This information was gathered from two websites: CMSI's website at www.travelrn.net/rnlicensure/FMPro and AMN's website at www.nursingmanagement.com/licensin.htm.

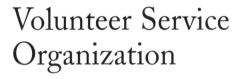

Volunteer Service Organization

Albert Schweitzer Institute Of the Humanities
P.O. Box 550
Wallingford, CT 06492-0550
203-697-3933
Locations: International

American Red Cross
Attn: Public Inquiry Office
431 18th Street, NW
Washington, DC 20006
202-639-3520
www.redcross.org
Locations: International

Association of Episcopal Colleges
815 Second Avenue, Suite 315
New York, NY 10017
212-716-6148
Location: International

Catholic Medical Mission Board
10 West 17th Street
New York, NY 10011-5765
212-678-5659
Locations: International

Christian Medical and Dental Society
P.O. Box 7500
Bristol, TN 37621
Location: Short term domestic
International mission trips

Church World Service
P.O. Box 968
Elkhart, IN 46515
800-297-1516
www.churchworldservice.org
Locations: International

Concern America
P.O. Box 1790
Santa Ana, CA 92702
800-CONCERN
www.churchworldservice.org
Locations: Central and South
America, Mexico, Mozambique

Cross Cultural Solutions
47 Potter Avenue
New Rochelle, NY 10801
800-380-4777
www.crossculteralsolutions.org
Locations: China, Cuba, Ghana
India, Peru

Friendship Bridge
3560 Highway 74, Suite B-2
Evergreen, CO 80439
303-674-0717
www.friendshipbridge.org
Locations: Guatemala, Vietnam

Global Health Council
1701 K Street, NW
Washington, DC 20006
202-833-5900
Locations: Africa, Asia, Caribbean, Latin America

Health Volunteers Overseas
P.O. Box 65157
Washington, DC 20035-5157
202-296-0928
www.hvousa.org
Locations: International

Helping Hands Health Education
948 Pearl Street
Boulder, CO 80302
888-241-0710
Locations: Africa, Nepal

Institute of Cultural Affairs
4750 North Sheridan Road
Chicago, IL 60640
773-769-6363
Locations: Africa, Asia, Central and South America, Europe

International Alliance for Children
2 Ledge Lane
New Milford, CT 06776
860-354-3417
Location: Manila

International Executive Service Corps
333 Ludlow Street
Stamford, CT 06902-8904
203-967-6000
www.iesc.org
Location: International

International Lifeline
Box 32714
Oklahoma City, OK 73123
405-728-2828
Location: Haiti

International Medical Corps
11 South 500 West Olympic
Boulevard, #506
Los Angeles, CA 90064-1524

International Voluntary Services
1000 Connecticut Ave., NW #901
Washington, DC 20036
202-387-5533
Locations: Bangladesh, Bolivia, Botswana, Caribbean, Ecuador,
Mali, Somalia, Zaire, Zimbabwe

Jesuit Volunteers International
P.O. Box 3756
Washington, DC 20007
202-687-1132
www.jesuitvolunteers.org
Locations: International

Maryknoll Lay Missioners
P.O. Box 307
Maryknoll, NY 10545-0307
800-818-5276
www.maryknoll.org
Locations: Africa, Asia, Latin America, U.S.

Mercy Corps International
3015 SW First Avenue
Portland, OR 97201
www.mercycorps.org
Locations: Africa, Americas, Balkans, East Asia, Middle
East/Caucasus, South and Central Asia

Operation Rainbow, Inc.
3760 Greenbriar
Stafford, TX 77477
877-810-7702
www.operationrainbow.org
Locations: Armenia, El Salvador, Guatemala, Mexico, Nicaragua,
Philippines, Venezuela, Vietnam

Pan American Health Organization
525 23rd Street, NW
Washington, DC 20037
202-974-3000
www.paho.org
Locations: International

Peace Corps
1111 20th Street, NW
Washington, DC 20526
800-424-8580
www.peacecorps.org
Locations: International

Project Concern International
3550 Afton Road
San Diego, CA 92123
858-279-9690
www.projectconcern.org
Locations: Bolivia, El Salvador, Guatemala, India, Indonesia,
Mexico, Nicaragua, Romania, U.S., Zambia

Project Hope
Health Sciences Education
Carter Hall
Millwood, VA 22646
540-837-2100
Locations: International

U.S. State Department
2201 C Street
Washington, DC 20520
202-647-4000
Locations: International

Volunteers for Mission
815 Second Avenue
New York, NY 10017
800-334-7626
Locations: International

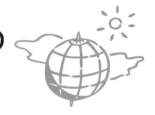

Staffing Agencies

Much of the information provided about the following agencies is relevant to the year 2001 and is subject to change. Several companies are in the process of changing and merging. You are provided here with the most accurate and current information possible. Much of the preliminary research has been done for you. Agency representatives were contacted by phone and by mail to update and confirm this information. Once the agencies realized a book was coming out for travelers, they were more than happy to participate. Occasionally, the responses to the standard questions were worded in such a way that the category had to be worded differently to reflect what was stated with better accuracy.

Regardless of the wording, each listing tells you when the company was founded, what kind of travelers they staff, what kind of housing is offered for free, and any benefits or information about the agency that makes them unique. Below each agency listing, space is provided for you to make personal notes, update any changes the agency has made, and note the name of your recruiter. This section can become your own personal handbook to refer to while traveling.

Advantage Nursing
American Nursing Services
Anestaff, Inc.
Australian Nursing Solutions
Catto International
CMSI
Cross Country Travcorps
Faststaff Nursing
Fidelity on Call, Ltd.
Geneva Health International
Health Care Everywhere
Health Staffers
Heartland Health Resources
HCCA International
Hospitalsupport
HRN Services
Kate Cowhig International

American Mobile Healthcare
American Traveler
Aramco Service Company
Bonnieville Health Recruiters
Clinical One
Core Medical Group
Elite Medical
Favorite Nurses
First Assist Travelers, Inc.
Gentiva Flying Nurses
Health Care Resource
    Management
Helen Zeigler & Associates, Inc.
Hospital Corp.
HPO Staffing
Intelistaf
Medical Express

Medical Staffing Network
Medstaff
NovaPro
Nurses RX
Nu-Tech Health Resources
Oxley Group
Preferred Health Care Staffing
Procare USA
Professional Resources for Nurses
Professional Staffing Resources
q-Shift Travel Nurses
Rapid Temps
RNNetwork
Specialty Professional Services
Stat Nursing Services
Surgical Associated Services
Surgical Staff
Surgistaff
Travel Nurse Across America
Travmed
World Wide Healthcare
    Exchange

Medsearch
Nannies Incorporated
Nurse Options USA
Nursing Management Services
O'Grady-Peyton International
PINS
Preferred Medical
Professional Recruiters/
    Temporary Resources
Psychiatric Care Consultants
    (PCC)
Resources on Call
RN Temps
Starmed Staffing Group
Sunbelt Staffing
Supplemental Health Care
Surgical Nurse
Team Staff
Travel Nurse International
TVL Healthcare

ADVANTAGE NURSING

3340 Severn Ave. #320
Metairie, LA 70002
800-749-1122
Fax 504-456-1144
www.AdvantageNursing.com

Staffing since: 1984

Travelers: RN, LPN, CST

Housing: Private

Notable: Claim to have the most luxurious housing

Name of Recruiter: _____

Personal Notes:

AMERICAN MOBILE HEALTHCARE

12235 El Camino Real #200
San Diego, CA 92130
800-282-0300
Fax: 800-282-0328
Contact@americanmobile.com
www.americanmobile.com

Staffing since: 1985

Travelers: RN, Nurse Managers, NP, RT, ST, Dialysis Tech.,
Radiology Tech., LVN/LPN, Pharmacist, CRNA, EEG Tech.,
Ultrasonographers, PT, PT assistant, OT, OT assistant, SLP,
Pulmonary Function Tech., Radiation Therapist, Polysomnography
Tech.

Housing: Private or shared, depending on the assignment

Notable: Professional and tenured recruiting staff

14,000 assignments in all 50 states

24-hour support

Name of Recruiter: _____

Personal Notes:

AMERICAN NURSING SERVICES

3012 26th St.
Metairie, LA 70002
800-444-6877
Fax: 504-837-2223
www.american-nurse.com

Staffing since: 1988

Housing: Private

Travelers: RT and PT (New Orleans area) and RNs statewide

Notable: Claim to have reputation for most desirable locations

Retention program

RN on call 24 hours a day, seven days a week

Name of Recruiter: _____

Personal Notes:

AMERICAN TRAVELER

1699 Federal Hwy. #300
Boca Raton, FL 33432
800-884-8788
Fax: 800-884-6510
Info@americantraveler.net
www.americantraveler.net

Staffing since: 1998

Travelers: RN, LPN, OT, PT, RT

Housing: Private; utilities included

Notable: U.S. and Canadian placement

Double overtime

CEU reimbursement

Can take 10 days off between assignments

Free AAA membership

Name of Recruiter: _____

Personal Notes:

ANESTAFF, INC.

4165 Shoreline Dr., Suite 15
Spring Park, MN 55384
877-ANESTAFF
Fax: 612-471-8898
mail@anestaff.com
www.anestaff.com

Travelers: CRNA, Anesthesiologist (MDA)

Name of Recruiter: _____

Personal Notes:

ARAMCO SERVICE COMPANY

P.O. Box 4530
Houston, TX 77210
Fax: 713-432-4600
Resumes@aramcoservices.com
www.jobsataramco.com

Staffing since: 1930

Travelers: Staff permanent RN positions

Housing: Private

Notable: 10 paid holidays

38 vacation days

4 travel days

One round trip to U.S. or Canada

Company-matched savings plan

Free health care in Saudi Arabia and optional group plan

Name of Recruiter: _____

Personal Notes:

AUSTRALIAN NURSING SOLUTIONS

25 Lansdowne Street
East Melbourne, Victoria 3002, Australia
+61 03 9662 9933
Fax: +61 03 9662 9933
ans@australiannursingsolutions.com.au
www.australiannursingsolutions.com.au

Travelers: RN

Housing: Subsidized

Notable: Staff in Melbourne, Australia, New Zealand, U.K.

Owned and operated by nurses

Monthly newsletter

Paid annual leave

Name of Recruiter: _____

Personal Notes:

BONNIEVILLE HEALTH RECRUITERS INC.
DBA PNS

1196 W. South Jordan Parkway, Suite C
South Jordan, UT 84095
800-777-6430
Fax: 800-541-8637
www.professionalnurse.com

Staffing since: 1975

Housing: Private/Shared

Travelers: RN, LVN, CST, LPN

Notable: Annual CE reimbursement

Tax advantage program

Have assignments nationwide in U.S., Virgin Islands, Guam

Name of Recruiter: _____

Personal Notes:

CATTO INTERNATIONAL LIMITED

75 Lynwood Dr.
Mytchett
Surrey GU16 6BU England
+44 1276 500 529
Fax: +44 1276 500 529
www.catto.net

Travelers: Doctors, nurses, pharmacists, veterinarians

Housing: Subsidized

Notable: Staff in U.K. and U.S.A.

Name of Recruiter: _____

Personal Notes:

CMSI

400 Randal Way #110
Spring, TX 77388
1-800-423-1739
Fax 800-253-1504
www.TravelRN.com

Staffing since: 1983

Travelers: RNs of all specialties

Housing: Private

Notable: Work only with independent contractors

Local check

Loans and advances

Cash advantage plan

Can take out quarterly taxes for you as a free service

Led the industry in using written contracts

Name of Recruiter: _____

Personal Notes:

CORE MEDICAL GROUP

Two Keewaydin Dr.
Salem, NH 03079
800-995-2673
Fax: 603-893-8442
Nurses@coremedicalgroup.com
www.coremedicalgroup.com

Staffing since (temporary staff): 1992

Travelers: Specialty RNs and LVNs (ICU/CCU, ER, OR, CST, Med/Surg, L&D, PED, NICU, Psych), OT, PT, Speech Pathologist

Housing: Shared

Notable: Claim their clients are some of the most prestigious medical institutions in the U.S.

Name of Recruiter: _____

Personal Notes:

CROSS COUNTRY TRAVCORPS

6551 Park of Commerce Blvd. N.W. #200
Boca Raton, FL 33437
800-343-3270
Fax: 800-803-1186
Info@cctc.com
www.crosscountrytravcorps.com

Staffing since: 1975

Housing: Free shared; other options involve a fee

Travelers: RN, ST, LPN, Case Management, Utilization Review,
Clinical Trials, RT, Radiological Techs., PT, OT, SLP, Medical Lab
Tech., Nurse Practitioners, CRNA, Clinical Nurse Specialist, Certified
Nurse Midwives, PA, Pharmacists

Notable: Largest medical staffing company in the nation

Large selection of assignments

Has a university to provide CEUs and professional development
opportunities

Name of Recruiter: _____

Personal Notes:

ELITE MEDICAL

100 Crescent Centre
Tucker, GA 30084
800-849-5502
Fax: 770-908-2203
Elitesearch.com
Info@elitesearch.com
www.elitemedical.com

Staffing since: 1992

Travelers: Radiology, RN

Housing: Private

Notable: Customized searches for desired location

Staff for temporary and permanent placement

Name of Recruiter: _____

Personal Notes:

FASTAFF NURSING

3888 E. Mexico Suite 123
Denver, CO 80210
800-736-8773
Fax: 800-743-6877
hiring@fastaff.com
www.fastaff.com

Staffing since: 1989

Travelers: RNs for all specialties, CNA, LVN, LPN

Housing: Shared, or pay 50% more for single

Notable: Claims to pay some of the highest rates

Long and short term (as little as 4 weeks)

Name of Recruiter: _____

Personal Notes:

FAVORITE NURSES

PO Box 7046
Shawnee Mission, KS 66207
800-755-1411
Fax: 800-882-8329
gotravel@favoritenurses.com
www.favoritenurses.com

Staffing since: 1981

Travelers: LPN, RN, CST

Housing: Private

Notable: Section 125 tax savings plan

AAA membership

CEU reimbursement up to 100 dollars per year

401(k) effective on first assignment

Name of Recruiter: _____

Personal Notes:

FIDELITY ON CALL, LTD.

PO Box 3597
Peoria, IL 61612-3597
800-836-7633
Fax: 309-691-8328
Fidelity@osc.link.com

Staffing since: 1994

Travelers: RN

Housing: Private

Notable: Staff in Midwestern U.S.

Name of Recruiter: _____

Personal Notes:

FIRST ASSIST TRAVELERS, INC.

4720 Montgomery Lane #300
Bethesda, MD 20814
800-426-1724
Fax: 301-718-2085
www.firstassisttravelers.com
info@firstassisttravelers.com

Staffing since: 1986

Travelers: RN, ST, Radiology Techs., RNFA, CFA

Housing: Private, furnished

Notable: Nurse owned and operated

Offices in DC, MD, OH, IL, TX, CA

Name of Recruiter: _____

Personal Notes:

GENEVA HEALTH INTERNATIONAL

Level 2
Hewlett Packard Building
137-147 Quay Street
Auckland
+64 9 916 0200
Fax: +64 9 916 0201
www.genevahealth.com
info@genevahealth.com

Travelers: RN, Physiotherapist, social worker, pharmacist

Notable: Staff in N.Z., U.K., Australia, Middle East, Canada, U.S.

Name of Recruiter: _____

Personal Notes:

GENTIVA FLYING NURSES

4101 McEwen Rd. #250
Dallas, TX 75244
800-950-3415
Fax: 800-677-4815
Info@flyingnurses.com
www.flyingnurses.com

Staffing since: 1980

Travelers: RN (ICU, TELE, MS, PED, NICU, ER)

Housing: Private

Notable: Bonus on every assignment

Weekly pay

License reimbursement each time

Name of Recruiter: _____

Personal Notes:

HEALTH CARE EVERYWHERE

4709A Eisenhower Ave
Alexandria, VA 22304
800-950-3345
Fax: 800-829-4906
www.Healthcareeverywhere.com

Staffing since: 1988

Travelers: PT, OT, SLP, Radiology, CST, RN

Housing: Private

Notable: Immediate health insurance

Tax-free per diem for meals

Name of Recruiter: _____

Personal Notes:

HEALTH CARE RESOURCE MANAGEMENT

P.O. Box 578
Cornelius, NC 28031
800-253-7131
Fax: 704-987-8866

Staffing since: 1985

Travelers: All RN specialties

Housing: Private

Notable: 24-hour support

VIP program bonus plan

Vacation pay after three assignments

Name of Recruiter: _____

Personal Notes:

HEALTH STAFFERS

5636 North Broadway
Chicago, IL 60660
800-621-1440
Fax: 773-561-3689

Staffing since: 1980

Travelers: Naval Medical Center, San Diego: RN's for NICU, PICU, Pediatrics, and Telemetry

The Tripler Army Medical Center, Honolulu: RN's in L& D, NICU, PICU, Pediatrics, Mother/Baby, Medical/Surgical, OR, Same-Day Surgery, PACU, and LPNs and ST in OR and L&D.

Housing: Shared

Notable: Claim you may work on any U.S. nursing license

Name of Recruiter: _____

Personal Notes:

HEARTLAND HEALTH RESOURCES

1302 1/2 Courthouse Ave.
Auburn, NE 68305
800-835-7248
Fax: 888-549-7246
info@hhrnurse.com
www.HHRnurse.com

Staffing medical professionals since: 1997

Travelers: RN, ST, Radiological Techs.

Housing: Private (including utilities)

Notable: 24-hour management access

1-week paid vacation after every two assignments

Company created by traveling nurses

First day life, vision, health, and dental coverage

Name of Recruiter: _____

Personal Notes:

HELEN ZEIGLER & ASSOCIATES, INC.

2403-180 Dundas St. West
Toronto, ON Canada M5G 1Z8
416-977-6941 or 800-387-4616 (within North America)
Fax: 416-977-6128
Hza@hziegler.com
www.hziegler.com

Staffing since: 1981

Travelers: RN (with 2-3 years of experience), RRT, Paramedics, Radiographers, MRI Techs., CT Techs., Medical Secretaries, Medical Transcriptionists, Doctors, Dietitians, PT, OT

Housing: Shared

Notable: Staff exclusively in Saudi Arabia and United Arab Emirates

Single status contracts

43-50 days vacation a year

1-2 year commitment required

Return airfare

Name of Recruiter: _____

Personal Notes:

HCCA INTERNATIONAL

222 2nd Avenue North
Nashville, TN 37201
800-932-4685
Fax: 615-255-7093
Usa@hccaintl.com
www.hccaintl.com

Staffing since: 1973

Travelers: RN, MD

Housing: Varies

Notable: Offices in TN, Canada, and Europe

Also staff 1-year contracts in Saudi Arabia at King Faisal Hospital

Name of Recruiter: _____

Personal Notes:

HOSPITALSUPPORT

8000 Anderson Square #112
Austin, TX 78757
877-932-7823
Fax: 888-551-9996
www.orsupport.com
Orsupport@jump.net

Staffing since: 1994

Travelers: All RN specialties and Allied Professionals including Radiologist, Pharmacist, CRNAs, First Assistants

Housing: Private

Notable: Office staffed by medical professionals

Offer profit sharing

Tax advantage program

Name of Recruiter: _____

Personal Notes:

HPO STAFFING

106 Chrystal Plaza Dr.
New Albany, MS 38652
800-611-6462
Fax: 513-891-6145
Crisisstaffing@healthpersonnel.com
hpo@healthpersonnel.com
www.healthpersonnel.com

Staffing since: 1987

Travelers: RN, LPN/LVN, ST, Laboratory Techs., Radiology Techs., RT

Housing: Private

Notable: Crisis staffing departments for 1 to 4 weeks and for long-term assignments

Name of Recruiter: _____

Personal Notes:

HRN SERVICES

8383 Wilshire Blvd. #258
Beverly Hills, CA 90211
800-476-5561
Fax: 323-951-7170
www.hrnservices.com

Staffing since: 1990

Travelers: LPN, RN, ST

Housing: Private

Notable: All RN recruitment staff

24-hour RN support

Offer an optional addition of cancer insurance

Name of Recruiter: _____

Personal Notes:

INTELISTAF

1000 South Rodney Parham
Little Rock, AR 72204
800-235-3134
Fax: 800-666-4077
Travel@Intelistaf.com
www.intelistaf.com

Travelers: RN, ST, PT, OT, Speech Therapist, RT, Pharmacist

Housing: Private

Notable: Take pride in professionalism and client satisfaction

Name of Recruiter: _____

Personal Notes:

KATE COWIG INTERNATIONAL

41 Dawson St.
Dublin 2 Ireland
353 (0) 1 671 5557
Fax: 353 (0) 1 671 5965
800-897-9587 from USA
cowhig@iol.ie

Staffing since: 1990

Travelers: RN, Radiographers

Housing: Subsidized

Notable: Placement in England, Ireland, Channel Islands

Owned and operated by a nurse

Free phone numbers from countries worldwide provided on web site

Name of Recruiter: _____

Personal Notes:

MEDICAL EXPRESS

357 South McCaslin Blvd. #100
Louisville, CO 80027
800-544-7255
Fax: 800-743-7257
info@medicalexpress.com
www.mymedex.com

Staffing since: 1985

Travelers: RN, Nurse Managers, NP, RT, ST, Dialysis Tech.,
Radiology Tech., LVN/LPN, Pharmacist, CRNA, EEG Tech.,
Ultrasonographers, PT, PT assistant, OT, OT assistant, SLP,
Pulmonary Function Tech., Radiation Therapist, Polysomnography
Tech.

Housing: Shared or private, depending on assignment

Notable: More than 14,000 openings in database

Many long-term incentives

Name of Recruiter: _____

Personal Notes:

MEDICAL STAFFING NETWORK

7100 East Belleview Ave. #302
Englewood, CO 80111
800-852-5257
Fax: 303-850-9519

Staffing since: 1988

Travelers: Focus is OR, CST

Housing: Private

Notable: Claim RN base salary no less than $22 an hour

Pet friendly

401(k) effective immediately

Immediate health insurance

Name of Recruiter: _____

Personal Notes:

MEDSEARCH

821 "N" St. #204
Anchorage, AK 99501
907-276-5707
Fax: 907-279-3731
Barb_s@akexec.com
www.akexec.com

Staffing since: 1983

Travelers: RN

Housing: Varies

Notable: Staff assignments in Alaska

Name of Recruiter: _____

Personal Notes:

MEDSTAFF INC.

297 S. Newtown Street Rd.
Newtown Square, PA 19073
800-732-9992
www.medstaffinc.com

Staffing since: 1987

Travelers: RN, LPN, ST, Radiology Techs., Therapist (Physical, Occupational, and Speech)

Housing: Private

Notable: Length of service reward program

Take pride in paying attention to details

Offices in CO, FL, CA (Los Angeles, San Francisco, and San Diego), Virginia, West Virginia, and Hawaii

Assignments in U.S. (including Alaska and Hawaii), Virgin Islands, Bahamas, Puerto Rico

Name of Recruiter: _____

Personal Notes:

NANNIES INCORPORATED

317 The Linen Hall
162-168 Regent St.
London W1B5TD
0044 207 437 8989
Fax: 0044 207 437 8889
nanniesinc@aol.com
www.nanniesinc.com

Staffing since: 1989

Travelers: Maternity nurses

Notable: Leading international nanny agency

Offices in London and Paris

Placements made worldwide

Name of Recruiter: _____

Personal Notes:

NOVAPRO

1408 Westshore Blvd
Tampa, FL 33607
888-668-2761
Fax: 813-282-9678

Staffing since: 1992

Travelers: OR RN, CST/ST, CRNA

Housing: Private (paid utilities and household items)

Notable: Market to your desired location

Pet friendly

Immediate health care coverage

Name of Recruiter: _____

Personal Notes:

NURSE OPTIONS USA

6542 Hypoluxo Road #294
Lake Worth, FL 33467
800-863-8314
Fax: 800-357-8684
www.healthjobsusa.com

Staffing since: 1990

Travelers: RN, Nurse Management Personnel

Notable: Largest health care personnel sourcing service in the U.S.

Employers are provided subscription to the company and receive a list of candidates. The hospitals are allowed to contract with you directly.

Primarily focus on permanent staffing

Name of Recruiter: _____

Personal Notes:

NURSES RX

9800 West Kincey Ave. #150
Huntersville, NC 28078
800-733-9354
Fax: 704-875-9227
info@nursesrx.com
www.nursesrx.com

Staffing since: 1981

Travelers: RN, Nurse Managers, NP, RT, ST, Dialysis Tech.,
Radiology Tech., LVN/LPN, Pharmacist, CRNA, EEG Tech.,
Ultrasonographers, PT, PT assistant, OT, OT assistant, SLP,
Pulmonary Function Tech., Radiation Therapist, Polysomnography
Tech.

Housing: Shared or private, depending on assignment

Notable: Take pride in individualized plans and benefits

Matching funds for 401(k) plan

Incentive programs for cash, trips, and discounts

Name of Recruiter: _____

Personal Notes:

NURSING MANAGEMENT SERVICES

2400 Herodian Way Ste 110
Smyrna, GA 30080
800-797-8707
Fax: 800-546-5616
www.gonms.com

Staffing since: 1984

Travelers: RN, RT, LPN, ORT

Housing: Shared

Notable: Agency managed by nurses

Name of Recruiter: _____

Personal Notes:

NU-TECH HEALTH RESOURCES

611 South Market St.
Rock Port, MO 64482
800-834-1872
Fax: 800-896-9475

Staffing since: 1998

Travelers: ST, RN

Housing: Private

Notable: Market to areas requested

Gives you a choice of pay rate options (get paid more per hour with a lower completion bonus, or vice versa)

Name of Recruiter: _____

Personal Notes:

O'GRADY-PEYTON INTERNATIONAL

532 Stephenson Ave. #100
Savannah, GA 31405
877-504-7794
info@ogpinc.com
www.ogpinc.com

Staffing since: 1981

Travelers: RN, Nurse Managers, NP, RT, ST, Dialysis Tech., Radiology Tech., LVN/LPN, Pharmacist, CRNA, EEG Tech., Ultrasonographers, PT, PT assistant, OT, OT assistant, SLP, Pulmonary Function Tech., Radiation Therapist, Polysomnography Tech.

Housing: Shared or private, depending on assignment

Notable: Place U.S. nurses in U.K., Ireland, Australia, Guam, New Zealand

Immediate enrollment in 401(k) plan

Name of Recruiter: _____

Personal Notes:

OXLEY GROUP

GPO Box 62
Brisbane Qld 4001
Australia
1 300 360 456
Fax: 61 73222 4888
www.oxleygroup.com.au
nursing@oxleygroup.com.au

Travelers: RN

Housing: Varies

Notable: Staff in Australia

Name of Recruiter: _____

Personal Notes:

PINS (PROFESSIONAL INDEPENDENT NURSING SERVICES, INC.)

5345 Wyoming Blvd. NE Suite 202
Albuquerque, NM 87109
888-799-7467
Fax: 505-823-6426
Info@pinsnational.com
www.Pinsnational.com

Staffing since: 1994

Travelers: RN, LPN

Housing: Private

Notable: Nurse owned and operated

Corporate gym membership

Completion bonuses based on performance

AFLAC Disability/Cancer/Cafeteria Plan

Prepaid legal services and a 401(k) plan

Offices in CO, NM, TX, WA, OK

Name of Recruiter: _____

Personal Notes:

PREFERRED HEALTH CARE STAFFING

100 W. Cypress Creek Rd. #750
Ft. Lauderdale, FL 33309
800-735-4774
travel@preferredhealthcare.com
www.preferredhealthcare.com

Staffing since: 1981

Travelers: RN, Nurse Managers, NP, RT, ST, Dialysis Tech., Radiology Tech., LVN/LPN, Pharmacist, CRNA, EEG Tech., Ultrasonographers, PT, PT assistant, OT, OT assistant, SLP, Pulmonary Function Tech., Radiation Therapist, Polysomnography Tech.

Housing: Private or shared, depending on assignment

Notable: More than 14,000 assignments

Immediate enrollment in 401(k) program

Name of Recruiter: _____

Personal Notes:

PREFERRED MEDICAL

601 S Metcalf Suite 100
Louisburg, KS 66053
800-552-6845
Fax: 913-780-1540
Recruiter@preferredmedplacement.com

Staffing since: 1989

Travelers: RN, LPN, ORT

Housing: Private

Notable: Pride in being personable

Tax advantage plan

Name of Recruiter: _____

Personal Notes:

PROCARE USA

1799 Farmington Ave.
Farmington, CT 06085
800-877-6785
Fax: 860-675-8488
www.procareusa.com
procare@procareusa.com

Staffing since: 1990

Travelers: RN (American and Canadian), LPN, ST

Housing: Private

Notable: Personalized support to their clients

Name of Recruiter: _____

Personal Notes:

PROFESSIONAL
RECRUITERS/TEMPORARY RESOURCES

220 East 3900 South Ste #9
Salt Lake City, UT 84107
800-748-5047
Fax: 801-268-9940
recruitr@icw.com

Staffing since: 1977

Travelers: RN

Housing: Private

Notable: Members of large global network of recruiting companies
with domestic and international opportunities

Name of Recruiter: _____

Personal Notes:

PROFESSIONAL RESOURCES FOR NURSES

PO Box 10156
Enid, OK 73706
800-427-8334
Fax: 800-332-4137
www.prntravelnurse.com
customerservice@prntravelnurse.com

Staffing since: 1997

Travelers: RN, LPN, ST, RT

Housing: Private

Notable: Pride in providing experienced nurses (require 2 years of experience)

Owned and operated by RNs

Medical, dental, and life insurance

Name of Recruiter: _____

Personal Notes:

PROFESSIONAL STAFFING RESOURCES

P.O. Box 15093
Savannah, GA 31416
800-752-5166
Fax: 877-754-5337
psrnurses@aol.com
www.psrnurses.com

Staffing since: 1978

Travelers: RNs in all departments

Housing: Private

Notable: Pride in individualized plans

Provide career counseling and opportunities for professional development

Name of Recruiter: _____

Personal Notes:

PSYCHIATRIC CARE CONSULTANTS (PCC)

A.B.N. 88 059 305 547
P.O. Box 373 Heidelberg Victoria 3084
+61 3 9459 9999
Fax: +61 3 9458 4788
pcc@pccnurses.com.au

Staffing since: 1992

Travelers: RN (general division 1) SENs (division 2) and Psychiatric Nurses (Division 1 and/or 3); Personal Care Attendants

Housing: Not provided

Notable: Largest supplier of casual and contract mental health staff in Australia

All nurses must have current registration with Victorian or NSW Nursing Boards.

Can also assist nurses to work in U.K.

Open 24 hours, 7 days a week

Name of Recruiter: _____

Personal Notes:

Q-SHIFT TRAVEL NURSES

214 E. Monument Street
Colorado Springs, CO 80903
800-733-6877
Fax: 888-633-2285
info@guardingcare.com
www.guardingcare.com

Staffing since: 1990

Travelers: RN, LPN, ORT, ST

Housing: Private

Notable: Generous bonuses, licensure and CEU reimbursement

Nontaxable weekly living expense

Flexible contracts

401(k) with company matching

Name of Recruiter: _____

Personal Notes:

RAPID TEMPS

PO Box 1200
Artesia, NM 88211
800-581-4846
Fax: 505-746-8979

Staffing since: 1990

Travelers: RN, Radiology, Lab, RT

Housing: Private

Notable: Vehicle subsidy or car rental option

Name of Recruiter: _____

Personal Notes:

RESOURCES ON CALL

PO Box 3918
Hickory, NC 28603
800-777-3899
Fax: 888-847-4605
www.resourcesoncall.com

Staffing since: 1988

Travelers: Radiology, Therapists, Ultrasound and Allied Health, RNs

Housing: Private

Notable: Pride themselves in supporting quality

Approach you as a long-term employee

Name of Recruiter: _____

Personal Notes:

RNNETWORK

1900 NW Corporate Blvd #410W
Boca Raton, FL 33431
800-866-0407
Fax: 800-359-8480
www.rnnetwork.com

Staffing since: 1997

Travelers: RN, LPN, CST, Radiology Technicians

Housing: Private and free deluxe housing

Notable: Immediate free medical and dental insurance

Immediate free life insurance and 401(k)

Life partner insurance and AFLAC supplement available

Tax advantage program

Staff in U.S., Virgin Islands, and U.K.

Double time for overtime on most assignments

Name of Recruiter: _____

Personal Notes:

RN TEMPS

P.O. Box 404
Wayne, PA 19087
877-767-8233
Fax: 800-227-5701
www.rntemps.com

Staffing since: 1987

Travelers: Allied Health, RN

Housing: Private, fully furnished with all amenities (dishes, linen, TV) plus cable, phone, utilities

Notable: Approach you as a full-time employee

Recruiters are medical professionals

No list of availabilities; rather, find your desired location

Name of Recruiter: _____

Personal Notes:

SPECIALTY PROFESSIONAL SERVICES

4324 Clearview Expressway
Bayside, NY 11361
800-641-9111
Fax: 718-225-9421
www.specialtyproserv.com
info@specialtyproserv.com

Staffing since: 1993

Travelers: RN, ORT, LPN, CNA

Housing: Provide a housing allowance

Notable: Claim to have some of the highest salaries

Agency created by CCU nurses

Staff per diem and travel nurses in NJ, NY, FL, and CT

Name of Recruiter: _____

Personal Notes:

STARMED STAFFING GROUP

35 New England Business Center #260
Andover, MA 01810
800-782-7633
Fax: 800-700-1338
www.StarMed.com

Staffing since: 1980

Travelers: RN (all specialties), Therapy (PT, PTA, OT, COTA, ST, RT), Radiology (all levels and specialties), Pharmacy

Housing: Private

Notable: Largest full-service healthcare staffing company in U.S.

Instant 401(k) with employer contribution

Instant health insurance coverage

Paid CEU

Foreign recruitment assistance and some international

VHA preferred business partner

Name of Recruiter: _____

Personal Notes:

STAT NURSING SERVICES

1545 Broadway
San Francisco, CA 94109
800-962-8678
Fax: 800-939-7828

Staffing since: 1980

Travelers: RN, CST, LVN

Housing: Private

Notable: Nurse owned and operated

Very detailed in placing people

Nurse available for 24-hour support

Name of Recruiter: _____

Personal Notes:

SUNBELT STAFFING SOLUTIONS

3450 East Lake Road Ste 206
Palm Harbor, FL 34685
800-659-1522
Fax: 727-787-5975
Info@sunbeltstaffing.com
www.sunbeltstaffing.com

Staffing since: 1988

Travelers: RN, LPN/LVN, PT, PTA, OT, COTA, SLP, ORT

Housing: Private

Notable: Pay for professional workshops and seminars

In-house computer support for questions about your personal computer

Staff in a variety of settings: hospitals, outpatient facilities, skilled nursing, rehabilitation centers, school systems

Name of Recruiter: _____

Personal Notes:

SUPPLEMENTAL HEALTH CARE

2829 Sheridan Drive
Tonawanda, NY 14150
1-800-543-9399
Fax 716-832-9399
www.travelnurses.com

Specialize in OR placement since: 1984

Travelers: RN

Housing: Private

Notable: Immediate retirement vesting

U.S. and international placement (London, England; Dublin, Ireland; Australia; New Zealand)

Nontraditonal options such as occupational health, psychiatric and correctional nursing

Name of Recruiter: _____

Personal Notes:

SURGICAL ASSOCIATED SERVICES

6825 E. Tennessee Ave. #407
Denver, CO 80224
800-686-0457
Fax: 303-355-3199
Info@surgicalassociated.com
www.surgicalassociated.com

Staffing since: 1978

Travelers: Operating Room staffing only (RN,CST, CFA)

Housing: Private (pay utilities, phone, cable)

Notable: Specialize in what they know best (OR)

Offer a completion bonus every assignment

Pet and family friendly

Require 2 years of experience

Immediate 401(k) and medical benefits

Name of Recruiter: _____

Personal Notes:

SURGICAL NURSE

425 W Capitol Ave. #1562
Little Rock, AR 72201
800-240-2526
Fax: 800-924-1433
www.surgicalnurse.md

Staffing since: 1999

Travelers: RNFA, OR RN, ICU/CCU, Telemetry, Med/Surg RN, ST, Cath Lab RN

Housing: Private

Notable: Immediate health insurance

Phone allowance

Extension bonuses and sign-on bonuses

Name of Recruiter: _____

Personal Notes:

SURGICAL STAFF

125 Town Park Dr. #3004
Kennesaw, GA 30144
800-996-0577
Fax: 877-SSI-TRAV
www.surgicalstaff.com
travel@surgicalstaff.com

Staffing since: 1979

Travelers: OR RN, CST, Radiology, PACU, CCU, Central Processing

Housing: Private

Notable: Nurse owned and operated

Tax advantage program

Name of Recruiter: _____

Personal Notes:

SURGISTAFF

1037 La Londe Lane
Napa, CA 94558
707-265-9180
Toll free: 800-603-6664
Bay Area: 415-332-4006
Fax: 707-265-9182
www.surgistaff.com
susan@jobstation.com

Staffing since: 1997

Housing: Private or shared, depending on location/preference

Travelers: OR, Med-Surg, Telemetry, ICU, CCU, NICU, PICU, L&D, Peds, Surgical Tech, X-ray Techs; nationwide.

Notable: 401K and insurance benefits available within 30 days of initial start date

Competitive Rates

Referral bonus program

Name of Recruiter: _____

Personal Notes:

TEAM STAFF

2 Northpoint Dr. #110
Houston, TX 77060
800-600-0374
Fax: 800-700-0374

Staffing since: 1982

Travelers: RN, Radiology and Allied Health, Diagnostic Imaging, Cath Lab, MRI, Ultrasound

Housing: Private

Notable: Offices in Texas and Florida

Name of Recruiter: _____

Personal Notes:

TRAVEL NURSE ACROSS AMERICA

425 W. Capitol Ave, Suite 1550
Little Rock, AR 72201
800-240-2526
Fax: 501-663-2886
www.nurse.tv
www.surgicalnurse.tv

Staffing nurses since: 1998

Travelers: RN

Housing: Private

Notable: Health insurance effective first day

Free 1300-minute calling card with each assignment

Can earn paid vacation time

Tax advantage program

Name of Recruiter: _____

Personal Notes:

TRAVEL NURSE INTERNATIONAL

703 Market Street #1212
San Francisco, CA 94103
1-800-249-5098
Fax: 877-822-6892
Hotline: 800-600-1432
contact@travelnurseinternational.com
www.travelnurseinternational.com

Staffing since: 1999

Travelers: RN

Housing: Shared

Notable: Staff strikes, crisis staffing, and long-term staffing

Expanding to international placement

Name of Recruiter: _____

Personal Notes:

TRAVMED

5250 77 Center Dr. #300
Charlotte, NC 28217
800-567-6944
Fax: 704-586-0623

Staffing since: 1996

Travelers: Radiology, RN, RT

Housing: Private

Notable: Tax advantage program

24-hour support

License reimbursement

Name of Recruiter: _____

Personal Notes:

TVL HEALTHCARE

11585 Jones Bridge Rd #420-226
Alpharetta, GA 30022
800-265-9363
Fax: 800-368-5161

Staffing since: 1996

Travelers: RN, CST

Housing: Private with washer/dryer

Notable: Weekly pay

Specialize in staffing operating rooms

Most assignments pay double time in overtime

Name of Recruiter: _____

Personal Notes:

WORLD WIDE HEALTH CARE EXCHANGE

The Clonnades
Beaconsfield Close
Hatfield
Hertfordshire AL108YD, UK
+44(0)1707 259233
Fax: +44(0)1707259233
Info@whe.co.uk
www.whe.co.uk

Staffing since: 1949

Travelers: Nurses, OT, PT, Physician, Pharmacist

Housing: Varies

Notable: Recruits candidates to U.K. from Australia, New Zealand, Canada, Philippines, Singapore, China, Europe

Recruits nurses to Australia, New Zealand, Canada, U.S.

Offices in Canada (info@whecan.com), Australia (healthcare@ melb.whe.com.au), New Zealand (whenz@nznet.gen.nz), U.K.

Good idea to plan 6 to 9 months in advance

Name of Recruiter: _____

Personal Notes:

Index

Page numbers followed by f indicate figure.

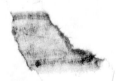